Breast Cancer Nursing
and Counselling

Diane J. Marks-Maran

BSc, SRN, DipN(Lond), FETC, RNT
Tutor, St Bartholomew's
Hospital, London

Barbara M. Pope

SRN
Formerly: Clinical Nurse Specialist,
Breast Unit, Royal Marsden
Hospital, London

FOREWORD BY

The Baroness Cox of Queensbury

Formerly: Director, Nursing
Education Research Unit,
Chelsea College, London

BLACKWELL SCIENTIFIC
PUBLICATIONS
OXFORD LONDON EDINBURGH
BOSTON PALO ALTO MELBOURNE

© 1985 by
Blackwell Scientific Publications
Editorial offices:
Osney Mead, Oxford, OX2 0EL
8 John Street, London, WC1N 2ES
23 Ainslie Place, Edinburgh, EH3 6AJ
52 Beacon Street, Boston,
  Massachusetts 02108, USA
744 Cowper Street, Palo Alto,
  California 94301, USA
107 Barry Street, Carlton,
  Victoria 3053, Australia

First published 1985

Set by Burns & Smith, Derby
Printed and bound by Butler &
Tanner Ltd, Frome, Somerset

DISTRIBUTORS

USA
  Blackwell Mosby Book Distributors
  11830 Westline Industrial Drive
  St Louis, Missouri 63141

Canada
  Blackwell Mosby Book Distributors
  120 Melford Drive, Scarborough
  Ontario M1B 2X4

Australia
  Blackwell Scientific Book
  Distributors
  31 Advantage Road, Highett
  Victoria 3190

British Library
Cataloguing in Publication Data

Marks-Maran, Diane J.
  Breast cancer nursing and
  counselling.
  1. Breast—Cancer 2. Cancer—
  Nursing
  I. Title II. Pope, Barbara M.
  616.99′449′0024613 RC280.B8
  ISBN 0-632-01024-X

Contents

     Metastatic Disease, 136

     Appendices

     1   The Mastectomy Association, 145

     2   Counselling Organisations, 146

     3   Directory of Apparel/Prostheses Suppliers, 147

     Index, 157

Foreword

This is an important and significant book. It is important because it can make a valuable contribution to the quality of nursing care for the many thousands of women with cancer of the breast. It is significant because it makes an addition to the growing body of literature which demonstrates that nursing is 'coming of age' professionally.

First and foremost, the book offers nurses relevant information which can help them to help women who have to go through ordeals associated with breast cancer: the inevitable shock and anxiety of being told the diagnosis; the subsequent treatment, which is inherently stressful and possibly mutilating; and the problems of living with the continuing knowledge of having been treated for a malignant disease. The book therefore provides nurses with a wide range of information relating to issues from physiology and chemotherapy to counselling and domiciliary care.

Secondly, it is important to stress that the book is written by nurses for nurses. Its style reflects this — it is generally down-to-earth, readable and, at times, colloquial. There are also aids for teaching and learning, such as questions at the end of chapters. But as well as being a useful 'reader' for practitioners, educators and students, this book is another indicator that nursing is 'coming of age' professionally, for it represents a synthesis of knowledge drawn from different disciplines, brought together in an attempt to enhance standards of nursing care. It thus adds to the growing body of nursing knowledge.

We can be grateful to the authors for making this knowledge more readily available, and the onus now lies with nurses to avail themselves of it and to use it in their own professional practice. Without such nursing-related knowledge — together with the application of that knowledge to nursing practice and in nursing education — any claims to professionalism are mere rhetoric. But with these developments, we can endeavour to move forward as 'the major caring profession' with integrity and with compassion, enhanced by practice rooted and grounded in research-based knowledge.

If the book succeeds in its objectives, it will achieve that goal which is of ultimate value: a contribution towards the alleviation of human suffering. It is for the attainment of this goal that I wish it every success.

The Baroness Cox

Preface

There is a great need for this book. Although the library shelves in most schools of nursing might have several books about breast cancer, if one looks closely at these one finds that they are written for two types of people: doctors and lay people. This book is a book for nurses and the focus is on nursing care and counselling. It is for all nurses — hospital and community — who, in the course of their careers, come across women with breast cancer needing good nursing care. It is written by nurses — nurses who have many years collective experience looking after women with breast cancer and who have come to realise that in many hospitals nurses are often not given enough information about breast cancer, implications of treatment, alternatives of treatment and how to meet these women's psychological needs. We believe that this book can help.

The book is divided into several sections. Chapter 1 sets the scene for the implications of breast cancer by discussing the normal, healthy breast and what it means psychologically, socially and anatomically. Chapters 2 and 3 introduce the subject of breast cancer by outlining the nature of the disease and what goes wrong in the cell growth to cause breast cancer, and how breast cancer is detected. Chapters 4 and 5 examine the role of surgery in breast cancer both in terms of primary surgical treatment and of breast reconstruction. Chapters 6 and 7 look specifically at care and counselling of women following mastectomy while they are still in hospital. These chapters deal with prostheses, advice about clothing and the particular counselling needs of hospitalised patients after breast surgery. Chapter 8 takes a close look at nursing care and counselling of patients with breast cancer when they return home and also at the facilities for support in the community. Rightly or wrongly, the majority of women with breast cancer in this country are treated with some form of surgical procedure. This is why this book begins with the nursing care related to surgery to the breast. Chapters 9,10 and 11, however, discuss in detail the role of radiotherapy, chemotherapy and hormone therapy in women with breast cancer, and the nursing and counselling implications of these treatments. The concluding chapters discuss local and systemic effects of breast cancer specifically related to the problems of lymphoedema and metastatic spread of breast cancer.

Although this book focusses upon nursing and counselling, we have gone into fairly great depth about cell growth, the kinetics of chemotherapy, cellular effect of radiotherapy and other aspects of breast cancer and its treatment. Our experiences have shown us that many nurses are ignorant about the physiological behaviour of cancer and how various forms of treatment actually work. We believe that without adequate knowledge of these things nursing care can become routine and meaningless and that nurses need a sound basis of knowledge both to anticipate problems which may arise from the illness and its treatment and to keep the patient informed and prepared for what to expect. We also believe that nurses often need guidelines on how they can offer practical advice and help to women with breast cancer. For this reason, Appendix 1 provides information about The Mastectomy Association, while Appendices 2 and 3 give lists of useful addresses to which both patients and nurses can turn for advice and information about breast cancer, alternative treatments, clothing and prostheses.

From an educational point of view we believe that this book provides teachers and charge nurses with valuable material for both ward and classroom teaching. Nearly every chapter has a teaching and learning exercise at the end which is related to that chapter. They are organised so that they can be used for individual reflection and study or for group work and discussion.

Chapters 7 and 8 are by Mimi Hondagneu and Sylvia Denton respectively. Mimi was a Clinical Nurse Specialist, in the Breast Unit, at the Royal Marsden Hospital and Sylvia is the Mastectomy Nurse at King's College Hospital. Both have been leaders in improving the care received by patients with breast cancer and their help, advice and expertise have been invaluable to us.

We believe that patients with breast cancer are not always aware of what they should expect when they seek treatment. Nurses must be aware and knowledgeable in order to provide the information, care and advice which these women need. We believe that this book can provide nurses with that awareness and knowledge.

Diane Marks-Maran
Barbara Pope

Acknowledgements

We would like to give thanks to the many people who supplied advice and information regarding their products, and were also kind enough to be willing to donate photographs when needed, namely Camillia Kennet of Remploy, Mr Rice of Spencer Banbury, Mrs Stewart of Torplay, Sheila Goodenough at Dow Corning, and the team at Camp Ltd.

Thanks also to Clyne Cullen and Mr and Mrs Kenton of Contour who were kind enough to give us their time and advice about suitable bras and swimwear and to Jobst UK, who supplied literature and photographs about lymphoedema treatment and care.

The Appendix on the Mastectomy Association could not have been written without the guidance of Iris Field, for which we are grateful. Personal thanks to David, Judith and Marian, without whom the enormous task of completing the manuscript would have been virtually impossible!

Lastly, our thanks to the many people who have taught us about *living* with cancer.

Chapter 1
The Breast in Health

Henry Gray describes the breasts as being: 'two large hemispherical eminencies situated toward the lateral aspect of the pectoral region, corresponding to the intervals between the 3rd and 6th or 7th ribs, and extending from the sternum to the axilla' (Gray 1973).

This clearly tells us where they are! The breasts are very small before puberty, but begin to develop under the influence of the female hormones. During pregnancy and lactation, a further increase in size can be seen, whilst after the menopause they atrophy.

Structure

The left breast is generally a little larger than the right, though no-one has yet offered a reason for this being so. They are separated from the underlying pectoral muscles by a layer of fascia. The nipple is situated just below the centre of the breast. The surface of the nipple, dark in colour, is surrounded by an areola which in a woman who has not borne children is described as being not dark but delicately deeper than skin tone. In the pregnant woman, the colour of the areola changes to a darker brown which increases as the pregnancy advances. The areola returns to its former size after lactation ceases, though it never regains its former colour.

The nipple is cylindrical in shape and is capable of erection from mechanical excitement (sexual stimulus, heat, cold) — a change which is mainly due to the contraction of its muscular fibres. It too, like the areola, has a brownish hue, and contains minute openings for the lactiferous ducts. Numerous sebaceous glands are found at the base of the nipple and on the surface of the areola. These glands become enlarged during lactation and secrete a fatty substance which lubricates and protects the nipples during breastfeeding. These are known as Montgomery's tubules, after the man who first described them.

1

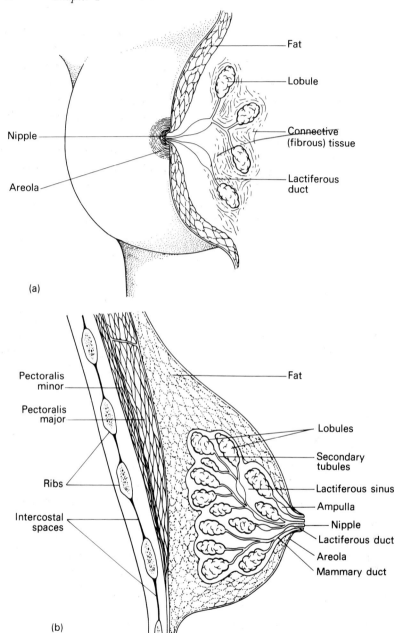

Fig. 1.1 Anatomy of the breast (a) and cross-section (b).

The mammary glands consist of glandular, fibrous and adipose tissue. Glandular tissue is composed of lobes, alveoli and ducts. There are approximately 20 lobes in each breast and each lobe is made up of lobules which consist of the alveoli. The alveoli open into smaller channels which in turn unite to form the lactiferous ducts. These ducts converge towards the centre of the breast behind the nipple where they dilate to form a lactiferous sinus. During lactation these sinuses will act as reservoirs for the milk. The duct finally constricts before reaching the nipple. The fibrous tissue encompasses the glandular tissue and forms the supporting suspensory ligaments (Cooper's ligaments are examples of such fibrous tissue and help to keep the breasts in position). The fatty tissue covers the surface of the breast tissue and occupies the spaces between the lobes. The amount of fat is proportional to the size of the breast (Fig. 1.1).

BLOOD SUPPLY

The breasts are supplied with blood from the thoracic branches of the axillary arteries and from the internal mammary and intercostal arteries. The venous return is described as an anastomotic circle around the base of the nipple and was called the *circulus venosus* by Haller. Branches from this carry blood to the circumference of the breast and end in the mammary and axillary veins.

LYMPHATIC SYSTEM

Much consideration is later given to the treatment and state of the lymphatic glands, therefore it is important we understand a little about their position and function in relation to the female breast (Fig. 1.2).

Superficial lymphatic glands may be found lying beside the cephalic vein between the deltoid and pectoralis major muscles (Fig. 1.3). Deeper set glands may be found in the axilla. They are fairly large in size and usually number 10–12. These glands form a chain which surrounds the axillary blood vessels and receives the lymphatic vessels from the arm. Remaining lymphatic glands are arranged in two small chains, the first one runs along the border of the pectoralis major, receiving the lymphatics from the chest and mammae, and

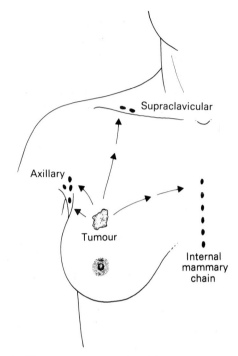

Fig. 1.2   Spread of breast cancer to regional lymph nodes.

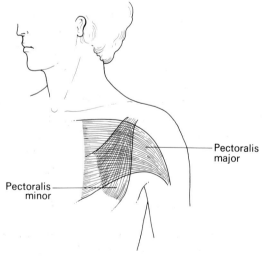

Fig. 1.3   Muscles surrounding the breast.

the second which lies along the posterior wall of the axilla, receiving the lymphatics from the back. Found immediately beneath the clavical are the subclavian or infraclavicular glands. The efferent vessels from the axillary gland accompany the subclavian vein into the neck and from there join the thoracic duct. The internal mammary chain is found beneath the sternum in the intercostal spaces.

Physiology

We have looked briefly at the anatomy of the female breast, now let us look at the physiology of the breast in health (Fig. 1.4). Manipulation of oestrogen and progesterone has a large part to play in the control and management of breast cancer and this will be discussed in more detail in Chapter 11. The development of breasts begins at puberty under the influence of oestrogen and progesterone. Pituitary function also needs to be normal. Each month the breasts respond to the varying levels of circulating hormones, and prepare themselves for a possible pregnancy. They become enlarged and engorged as the glands grow, and this is part of the reason for the 'lumpiness' and soreness that many women feel prior to menstruation.

The onset of the menopause will occur as the ovary produces less oestrogen; however, circulating levels of oestrogen can still be found in smaller quantities because the adrenal gland produces this hormone in small amounts. Because of the diminished level of oestrogen, the breasts atrophy and are no longer subjected to cyclical changes. Breasts of menopausal ladies change in a few ways: during the 40s to 50s the amount of glandular tissue gradually diminishes and is replaced by fibrous tissue and fat (especially if 'middle age spread' is evident). As they reach their 60s and 70s the fat is generally lost, and so the breasts droop and the skin becomes wrinkled.

Social and cultural attitudes

But what of the cultural importance of breasts? We know where they are, what they do and how they work, but why do our breasts seem so important? It has been said that we live in a breast-orientated

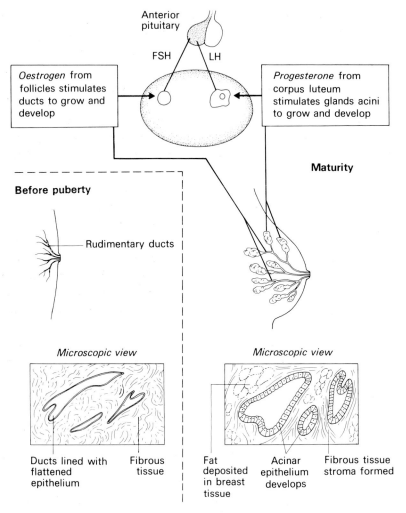

Anterior pituitary

FSH   LH

Oestrogen from follicles stimulates ducts to grow and develop

Progesterone from corpus luteum stimulates glands acini to grow and develop

Maturity

Before puberty

Rudimentary ducts

Microscopic view

Microscopic view

Ducts lined with flattened epithelium

Fibrous tissue

Fat deposited in breast tissue

Acinar epithelium develops

Fibrous tissue stroma formed

Fig. 1.4 The development of the breast in health.

society. Today's advertising methods indicate that breasts, uncovered or almost covered, can sell anything from cars to suntan oil. Films, billboards and magazines all indicate that large, firm, rounded breasts are a sexual and desirable asset. Since the 1940s, when Hollywood provided the public with female sex symbols with their hour-glass figures, voluptuous bosoms have been in fashion.

It is a little wonder that many women are led to believe that their bosom is less than perfect, and spend millions of pounds each year on bras to make their bosoms look bigger, smaller, more rounded, more cleavaged, etc., whilst more money is spent on creams and plastic surgery. All this has a lasting effect on a young girl as she reaches puberty and begins to develop breasts. Freudian analysts would maintain that breasts are a late consolation prize for not having a penis! Many other psychologists suggest that the young girl will compare her firm youthful bust with that of her mother's and that this would lead to feelings of guilt.

Girls often hide their developing breasts away from their fathers. Apparently the reason for this is twofold: first, many girls are going through a stage in which their fathers are becoming attractive to them as males (Electra complex), and second, this leads them to feel that they are in direct competition with their mother for their father's attention. At this stage many girls become confused and anxious about their awakening feelings and may put off buying a bra, and wear constricting or baggy clothes which hide their developing breasts from the world.

At some point she will realise whilst exploring her own body, that her breasts can be a source of distinct pleasure. Most girls go through a phase of allowing other girls to touch their breasts at some time during their sexual development. This would seem to be a normal practice which precedes a heterosexual relationship. Once she notices boys are interested in her shape, she will start to buy bras and clothes which will enhance what 'mother nature' has given her.

The shape of the fully developed bosom is unique from one woman to the next, but there are certain 'types' which are hereditary to some degree and can be modified only slightly by the owner. British women fall into two distinct categories: small-backed and large-bosomed, or wide-backed and small-bosomed, with both types varying in the amount of fat present.

As nurses we are also health educators and have many opportunities throughout our professional life to discuss with our female patients sensible ways of caring for a healthy breast; some examples of care are:

1   Always wear a sensible bra, especially if you are large-breasted.

2 Exercises will not make the breasts any larger, however it will give them a better shape.

3 Correct posture also enhances a woman's figure.

4 Massaging specialised creams onto the breast is not thought to influence their size.

5 Monthly checks of the breasts are advisable so that any abnormalities may be dealt with swiftly.

REFERENCE

Gray, H. (1973) *Gray's Anatomy,* p. 1038, 35th edn. Longman Group Ltd, Harrow, Essex.

FURTHER READING

Andrew & Stanway, P. (1982) Breasts in Society. In *The Breast.* Granada Publishing, London.

Andrew & Stanway, P. (1982) The Breast at Special Times of Life. In *The Breast.* Granada Publishing, London.

Ross, J. & Wilson, K. (1968) Reproductive System. In *Foundations of Anatomy & Physiology,* 3rd edn. Churchill Livingstone, Edinburgh.

Chapter 2
The Nature of Breast Cancer

To understand the nature of breast cancer it is necessary to understand the nature of normal cell growth and then to explore what happens to cells when cancer occurs.

Normal cell growth

Human growth occurs in two stages. The first stage takes place from conception to adulthood where the main purpose of growth is to increase the number of cells as the human being grows larger. The second stage occurs from adulthood until death when the main purpose of growth is so that the individual cells and tissues may continue their functions. As cells are lost, more are produced to replace them rather than to increase their total number. In adulthood, some tissues reach their total maximum cell numbers at maturity and for the rest of the individual's life are slowly but constantly wearing out. The cells of the nervous system are examples of these. In other tissues, however, cells are constantly proliferating to replace lost or dead cells. Examples of these are skin cells, blood cells and cells of the intestinal lining.

Normal human cell growth and behaviour are regulated by certain physiological controls which govern how much cell growth takes place and when this growth will occur. Each cell knows, through its chemical structure, what its unique function is, how much of the nutrient supply from the blood it needs to function, when and how to reproduce and when to mature and die.

Cancer cell growth

Cancer cell growth occurs when a single cell stops exhibiting one or more of the physiological controls which regulate its growth.

Although there is no one reason why this happens it is thought to occur due to either outside (exogenous) factors (carcinogens) such as smoking, and asbestos, or to endogenous or innate factors, like hormones or other body chemicals. In any event, an individual cell escapes from the physiological mechanisms governing cell growth and begins to grow in an uncontrolled manner. As the tumour grows in size it resembles the tissue in which it arose less and less. The degree to which a tumour resembles and behaves like its parent tissue is called *differentiation*. Types of tumour differentiation will be explained later in this chapter.

This chapter is not intended to provide a complete explanation of the dynamics of cell growth and reproduction. The subject of cell division and reproduction can be treated as an entire chapter on its own. Several excellent books are available which will help nurses to understand more about the intricacies of cell growth and behaviour and details of these and other suitable reading material are included at the end of the chapter.

The cell cycle

Prior to 20 or 30 years ago it was believed that cell reproduction (mitosis) was a continuous process with short rest periods in between. It is now known that mitosis takes place in a fairly short space of time. Before mitosis takes place the genetic material in the nucleus of the cell (DNA) replicates into two new strands so that the new cells which are to be formed will have the same characteristics as the old cell. Once this has happened, mitosis can take place. It is now also known that some cells which are expected to undergo mitosis may not be dividing at all for a certain period of time. In other words, some cells at any given moment may be 'resting' for various lengths of time rather than getting ready to divide and reproduce, being in the actual process of reproducing or having just completed their reproductive phase. This led to the formation of the concept of the *cell cycle* (Fig. 2.1).

In Fig. 2.1, G_1 represents a fairly dormant phase where the cell is gathering energy to ready itself for DNA replication (splitting of the strand of genetic material in the nucleus to form two, new identical cells).

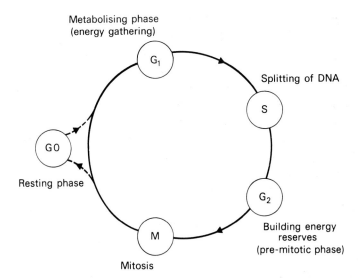

Fig. 2.1   The cell cycle.

The S phase represents the synthesis phase where the genetic material in the nucleus (DNA) actually splits and forms two new strands.

The G_2 phase is a second fairly dormant phase where the cell is gathering energy to enable it to undergo cell division.

The M phase is where mitosis (cell division) takes place.

The reader will also see in the diagram a phase which is labelled G_0. This is the phase which represents that time when certain cells are resting and are not dividing, getting ready to divide or recovering from recent cell division. These cells are said to be temporarily removed from the cell cycle but with the right stimulation they will return into the cell cycle to undergo cell reproduction.

Further implications of the cell cycle will be discussed in relation to chemotherapy in Chapter 10. The preceding information has been used to introduce the subject of the nature of breast cancer because, without this basic understanding of normal cell growth and division, it is often difficult to really understand what has gone wrong with cell growth to cause cancer to arise.

This has been only a brief overview of cell growth and reproduction. It is fairly widely believed that it is during DNA replication or mitosis that some change in normal cell activity occurs to cause cancer.

TYPES OF MALIGNANCY

Duct adenocarcinoma

Malignant change can arise in any part of the breast. The most common of the breast cancers, however, are those which arise in the ducts of the breast (*see* Fig. 1.1). Tumours which arise within a duct and do not grow outside the duct are known as *intraduct adenocarcinomas*. These tumours are preinvasive. Tumours which arise within the duct but spread to tissue outside the duct are known as *invasive adenocarcinomas* or *infiltrating intraduct carcinomas*. Another name given to these tumours is scirrhous carcinomas from the Greek word *skleros* which means hard. The majority of breast cancers are duct carcinomas. Baum (1981) has indicated that 90% of all malignant breast tumours are invasive duct adenocarcinomas. It is therefore expected that the majority of patients with breast cancer with whom nurses will come into contact will have invasive duct adenocarcinomas.

Lobular carcinomas

Malignant changes in the lobules of the breast are relatively uncommon. Lobular tumours which remain within the affected lobule are preinvasive and are termed *lobular carcinoma in situ*. A lobular tumour which spreads outside the affected lobule is called a *lobular invasive carcinoma*. Lobular tumours are often associated with invasive or preinvasive changes either elsewhere within the same breast or in the opposite breast.

Sarcomas

Extremely rare tumours are breast sarcomas which arise within the connective tissue.

Secondary tumours

Breast tumours secondary to cancer elsewhere in the body are also rare malignancies which arise as metastatic spread.

HOW TUMOURS GROW

Like all malignancies, tumour growth is measured in terms of *cell doubling time*. Doubling time can be defined as the amount of time it takes for the cells in a tumour to double in number; it is measured on a logarithmic scale which relates the number of doublings to the number of cells present in the tumour (Fig. 2.2).

One of the difficulties in detecting and treating tumours is that, by the time the tumour is first palpable (approximately 1 cm in size), it has undergone about 30 doublings and contains about 10^8 cells (100,000,000 cells). Most breast cancers are even larger than this

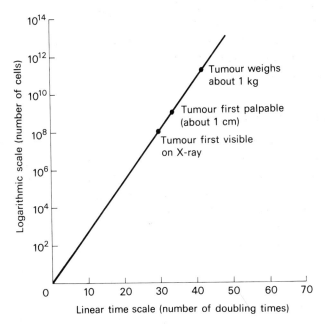

Fig. 2.2 Doubling time in relation to tumour size and detectability.

when first discovered; they have therefore undergone a greater number of doublings and contain more malignant cells. This problem is compounded in our society by the fact that many women who find a lump in their breast are often too frightened of the possible consequences to seek immediate medical attention in the naive hope that perhaps it will go away.

Local spread

With many women, a lump in the breast will be the only presenting symptom. An invasive carcinoma, however, can cause other noticeable changes in the appearance of the breast.

NOTICEABLE CHANGES

If the tumour infiltrates along the lines of Cooper's ligaments, the skin overlying that ligament is pulled downwards causing a visible *dimple* to appear in the breast. This dimple is a characteristic of an invasive carcinoma (Fig. 2.3).

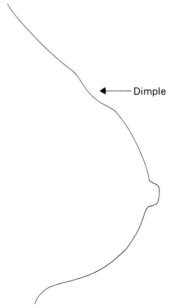

Fig. 2.3 Dimpling in skin caused by Cooper's ligaments being pulled downward by underlying tumour.

An invasive carcinoma can also invade along the lactiferous ducts (*see* Fig. 1.1). As the ducts shrink due to this invasion, the nipple is pulled inward — a phenomenon known as *nipple inversion* (Fig. 2.4).

As the tumour invades further into the breast it may become fixed to the skin overlying the breast, to the pectoralis major muscles or even to the ribs. Tumours which affix themselves to the skin often spread through the skin layers causing the skin to break down necrose and fungate. Some fast growing tumours can go unnoticed as lumps and first present as fungating lesions.

A tumour which infiltrates into a wide area of the breast can also cause excess fluid (oedema) in the skin overlying the tumour. The skin thickens in these areas and small dimples can occur in several Cooper's ligaments in the area. This gives the skin of the breast an orange peel appearance (often called 'peau d'orange').

Breast adenocarcinomas can also spread to local lymph glands and into the systemic lymphatic system. The axillary glands are the most common glands to be affected since the majority of breast tumours arise in the upper and outer quadrant of the breast. It is this

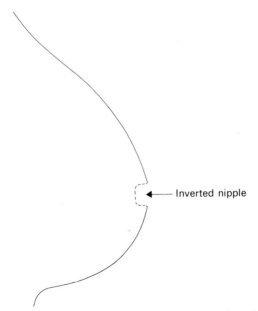

Fig. 2.4   Inverted nipple. Nipple is drawn inwards due to invasion of lactiferous ducts by the tumour.

area of the breast which drains lymphatic fluid into the axillary glands (*see* Fig. 1.2).

HOW IS BREAST CANCER STAGED ?

Breast cancer is staged in two ways — clinically and histologically.

Clinical staging

Clinical staging is carried out in terms of the size of tumour on palpation, whether or not lymph nodes can be palpated, and absence or presence of clinical signs of distant metastases. The Union Internationale Contre le Cancer has devised a means of staging breast cancer which is called TNM staging (UICC 1978). 'T' refers to tumour size/description, 'N' refers to size/description of nodes if present, and 'M' refers to absence or presence of distant metastases. Table 2.1 explains the TNM staging for breast cancer and is compared with the traditional method of staging breast cancer known as the Manchester system.

If a woman presents with a breast tumour which is staged as:

T 2a, N 1, M O

this means that the tumour is between 2 and 5 cm in size, that there are axillary nodes palpable but which are not fixed to the skin, and that there is no evidence of distant metastases. It is only by undertaking a full clinical staging like this that medical staff can make the best decision regarding the most appropriate way to treat a patient. This will be further outlined in later chapters which discuss the various ways of treating breast cancer.

Histological staging

The microscopic appearance of breast cancer can be examined in two ways. Firstly, cells can be aspirated from the tumour and examined to detect whether or not cancer cells are present. This is a diagnostic procedure and will be discussed in greater depth in Chapter 3.

Histological staging of breast cancer takes place after a sample of the malignant tissue has been removed following biopsy, excision of

Table 2.1   TNM staging to breast cancer.

Tumour

T 0	No palpable tumour
T 1	Tumour 2 cm or less with no fixation
T 1a	No attachment to underlying muscles
T 1b	Attached to underlying muscles
T 2	Tumour more than 2 cm but less than 5 cm with no fixation
T 2a	No attachment to underlying muscles
T 2b	Attached to underlying muscles
T 3	Tumour more than 5 cm in diameter
T 3a	No attachment to underlying muscles
T 3b	Attached to underlying muscles
T 4	Tumour of any size with either skin ulceration or fixation to chest wall

Nodes

N 0	No palpable axillary nodes
N 1	Palpable axillary nodes not fixed to skin
N 1a	Palpable axillary nodes not considered to contain tumour
N 1b	Palpable axillary nodes thought to contain tumour
N 2	Nodes greater than 2 cm or fixed to one another and to deep structures
N 3	Supraclavicular nodes involved

Metastases

M 0	No distant metastases
M 1	Distant metastases obvious

the lump or after more extensive surgery, such as wide excision or mastectomy. Pathologists prepare slides of the sample of tissue which is to be staged and examine the tissue microscopically to determine the extent of cell differentiation (*see* p.10 for definition).

Cancer cells can exhibit a wide variety of differentiation. At one end of the spectrum are those tissue specimens which contain recognisable tubules and ducts formed by the cancer cells which maintain similar characteristics to normal breast tissue. These tumours are called *well differentiated* tumours because of the close resemblance between them and normal breast tissue. At the other end of the spectrum are *poorly differentiated* and *anaplastic* breast cancers. Poorly differentiated tumours are those in which the cancer cells are practically unrecognisable as arising from breast tissue. Anaplastic tumours are those which are totally unrecognisable as arising from breast tissue.

The degree of differentiation appears to determine overall prognosis of the disease, with well differentiated tumours having the best prognosis.

TUMOUR GRADE

Differentiation is determined by ascertaining the *grade* of the tumour and this grade enables medical staff to have a fairly reliable understanding of prognosis of the disease and subsequent treatment. Grading is usually recorded as grades I, II and III. Occasionally, grade IV is also used.

Grading is determined by a point system, with points being given for the number of tubules seen microscopically, the state of the cell nuclei, and the mitotic activity. A well differentiated tumour with lots of recognisable tubules would be given one point. A moderately differentiated tumour with some recognisable tubules would be given two points and a poorly differentiated or anaplastic tumour with no recognisable tubules would be given three points. In terms of description of cell nuclei, one point is given if the majority of the nuclei are uniform, two points are given if many of the nuclei are uniform, and three points are given if the nuclei are totally nonuniform. Mitotic activity is also graded on a three point scale. By adding up the points for each of the three categories a histological grade is determined. Tumours with a total of 3–5 points are said to be grade I tumours. Those with a total of 6–7 points are called grade II tumours and those with a total point value of 8–9 points are said to be grade III tumours. The grade I tumours generally carry the better prognosis.

Because of the wide variety of ways in which breast tumours develop and grow and the wide varieties of histological presentations, breast cancer can not be viewed as one disease. It is, rather, a collection of diseases. No two tumours will act in the same way and it is only through individualised complete clinical and pathological staging that medical staff can plan individualised treatment for each woman.

HOW DOES BREAST CANCER SPREAD ?

Local spread to underlying tissue and overlying skin as well as invasion into the local lymph nodes are two ways in which breast cancer can spread. A third mode of spread is by cells or clumps of cells breaking off the original tumour and spreading to distant parts of the body via the bloodstream or the lymphatic system. It was mentioned previously that lymph nodes adjacent to the breast (such as in the axilla) are often the first place of spread. From these local lymph nodes, tumour cells can enter the general lymphatic circulation. Tumours in parts of the breast other than the upper and outer quadrant can spread to other local lymph nodes such as those in the supraclavicular region or in the internal mammary chain (*see* Fig. 1.4). The most common places for breast cancer to metastasize are the bones, liver, lungs and brain (Fig. 2.5).

SUMMARY

This chapter has attempted to describe the nature of normal cell growth and how cancer cells differ from normal cell activity. The nature of breast cancer has also been described. The authors firmly believe that nurses need an understanding of these basic facts and concepts in order to understand and recognise the problems and symptoms which arise in patients with breast cancer. This allows nurses to be more informed about what care they are giving and what needs may arise in patients. The most important points to iterate are:

1   Breast cancer is not one disease but a series of diseases.

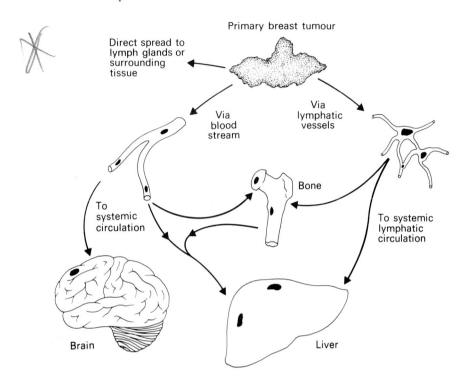

Fig. 2.5   How breast cancer spreads.

2   Because of this, nurses must realise that all patients will *not* progress in the same way nor will their disease spread in the same way.

3   Consequently, not all patients with breast cancer will respond in the same way to any given treatment.

4   If one patient does not respond to one type of treatment (be it surgery, radiotherapy, chemotherapy or hormone therapy) it does *not* follow that any other patient will not respond to that treatment. One can never generalise and say, for example, that mastectomy is totally useless merely because one patient was not cured. The same is true for the other forms of treatment. Each patient must be assessed individually and the outcome of treatment viewed only for that patient.

5   A good background knowledge of the nature of breast cancer will enable nurses to better understand why physicians and surgeons choose a particular course of treatment for their patients.

6   Good background knowledge also enables nurses to have the right information to advise and teach patients, relatives and other nurses about breast cancer and the various possibilities regarding treatment.

EXERCISE

Katherine is a 36-year-old air hostess for a British based airline. She has been married for six years and has one child, Simon, who is four-years-old. During the day Simon is looked after by Katherine's mother who lives nearby. Katherine has routinely been examining her breasts each month and during one such examination she discovered a lump in her left breast. She went to see her GP who referred her to the outpatient department of the local District General Hospital.

1   What investigations are likely to be carried out?

2   You are the nurse in the outpatient department. How would you explain these investigations to Katherine and prepare her for them?

REFERENCES

Baum, M. (1981) *Breast Cancer: The Facts.* Oxford University Press.

UICC (1978) *TNM Classification of Malignant Tumours,* UICC, Geneva.

FURTHER READING

Cobb, L. M. (1978) The Cancer Cell. In *Oncology for Nurses and Health Care Professionals,* R. Tiffany (ed.). Allen & Unwin, London.

Priestman, T. J. (1980) *Cancer Chemotherapy: An Introduction.* Montedison Pharmaceuticals, Barnet.

Chapter 3
Detecting Breast Cancer

Although as many as 12,000 women die each year from cancer of the breast, there are remarkably few screening units throughout the UK. Many hospitals have no access whatsoever to any screening methods, yet have to continue treating their patients. It is believed that if breast cancer is to be cured, then the chances of doing so increase the earlier it is detected. The purpose of screening asymptomatic women is to detect cancer earlier, so that less complicated treatment will be required to eradicate the disease, and the mortality rates should decrease. Screening usually consists of physical examination of both breasts, mammography, thermography, and instruction and encouragement to enable the woman to perform Breast Self Examination (BSE).

Breast self examination

When it comes to detecting breast cancer, no method can be more meritorious then Breast Self Examination. It costs nothing, does not entail any danger, and with correct teaching by the medical profession, it does not need an expert to perform it, and it can be done in privacy.

About 90% of all breast cancer symptoms are discovered by the woman herself or her sexual partner and are either accidental discoveries or as a result of BSE. Learning how to do BSE should be the responsibility of both the woman and health workers. Every effort should be made to provide an opportunity for each woman to learn the art of BSE at such places as postnatal clinics, family planning clinics, and during health check-ups with her GP. If these health workers do not initiate or encourage instruction, the woman may not feel happy to request it.

The basis of BSE is that after each monthly check, any change in the appearance, 'feel' or function of the breast is reported at once to her GP. Further examination by a specialist is desirable, in order to ascertain the nature of the abnormality. Why then, if it is so simple, do many women not avail themselves of this method of examination? There are many reasons given for not doing BSE. Some women do not like the thought of 'feeling themselves', others do not understand what they are feeling when touching their breasts, and mistake normal breast tissue and ribs for lumps. They either give up because they are frightening themselves, or make endless monthly visits to their GP. Many simply bury their heads in the sand, with the attitude that 'it won't happen to me, or if it does there is nothing I can do about it'.

It is important that adequate instruction should be given on how to perform this examination. Various leaflets are published which are designed to aid nurses in teaching women. The address at which these leaflets may be obtained are listed in Appendix 2.

Mammography and xeroradiography

Although the technology between mammography and xeroradiography is quite different, they both achieve a similar end product of a view of the soft tissue of the breast, so that, for the woman undergoing these tests, the instructions are the same. Mammography is the process of X-raying the soft tissue of the bosom; the end product is a mammogram (Fig. 3.1). Xeroradiography is also an X-ray of the bosom but the processing and results are different. In the latter, a metallic plate which has been charged with electricity is placed under the bosom. The X-ray which is then performed alters the pattern of the electrical charge on the plate, which is then developed by using a fine plastic powder. The finished result is a bluish film or photograph.

It is important to inform the woman of the procedure of mammography, as the machines used can look quite imposing. You could also tell her that usually two views of each breast, cranio caudal and lateral, are taken. A simple explanation may take the form of:

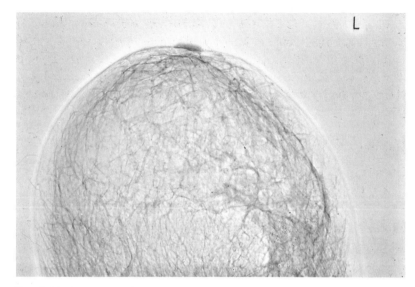

Fig. 3.1   A mammogram.

'Your doctor has requested a specialised X-ray of your bosom in order to help him diagnose you correctly. You will need to strip to the waist, and sit/stand in front of a machine. Your breasts, one at a time, will be gently placed on a ledge under which is an X-ray plate. A small dose of radiation is passed through the bosom onto the plate. The breast is kept in place on the ledge by gentle pressure from the top half of the machine. It should not hurt, nor be more than slightly uncomfortable. Once completed, you will be asked to wait until the films have been developed (a few minutes). If all views are of satisfactory standard, you can get dressed. The whole procedure should last no more than 10–15 minutes.'

Because of the use of radiation, women who are pregnant should not be submitted to this test except under extreme circumstances. Up-to-date mammographic techniques deliver as little as 0.5 rad (0.05 gray), but the unknown consequences of accumulated dosages, no matter how small, must be taken into account. This question about radiation may arise from the woman herself, especially if she is subjected to repeated tests of this nature.

The accuracy rates of mammography in detecting lumps are in the order of 95%. Younger breasts which have more glandular tissue tend to be a little more difficult to interpret than those of the middle-aged woman. Cancer is thought to be present if the mammogram shows an ill-defined opacity, minute calcifications, an increase in vascularity or enlarged lymph nodes.

Thermography

Thermography is a newer technique which measures the temperature of the skin over the breast. The test is used because it was found that some cancers of the breast gave out more heat than the surrounding tissues, a difference of 1–2°C is quite common. Again, careful explanation is needed.

'In this test, we will be taking a photograph of your bosom. You will be asked to undress to the waist and sit in a small waiting room on your own, with your arms raised. The room is set at a cool constant temperature (approximately 20°C, 68°F). After about 10 minutes you will be asked to go into an adjoining room where your breasts will be photographed, using an infra-red camera. Three different views are taken and this records the skin temperature. The whole procedure takes about 15 minutes, and does not hurt in any way. When the photographs have been taken you will be free to go.'

The heat-loss from the skin is recorded on film and the different densities denote corresponding heat-loss. The drawback of using this method of detection is that it is not very reliable. It rarely detects more than 70–85% of cancers, and can give a false positive result in 15–40% of cases (Moskowitz *et al.* 1976). Not all cancers produce a heat-detectable pattern, and it has also been shown that scratches, insect bites/stings, and even bronchitis can produce a misleading picture. For these reasons, thermography results are used only in conjunction with other diagnostic tests.

Ultrasound

Ultrasound is another painless noninvasive test. It is at present an untested and time-consuming method of detecting breast cancer. Ultrasound involves passing high-frequency sound-waves through the breast and building up a picture of the waves as they bounce back from the internal structures. As yet techniques vary considerably, so it is up to each nurse to familiarise herself with the particular method used in her unit. Ultrasound used in the detection of breast cancer still has a long way to go before it becomes widely used, but because of its simplicity, coupled with recent advances in technology, it should have a part to play in the near future.

Nuclear magnetic resonance

Nuclear magnetic resonance is a diagnostic method which is still in its infancy. The attraction is that no radiation is used. It endeavours to show up the differing densities of breast tissue but, as yet, no proof of its validity exists (Bovee & Getreuer 1978).

Routine breast screening

How effective is routine breast screening? According to a trial conducted in Edinburgh between 1975 and 1977, as many as 5 new cases of cancer per 1,000 women were discovered using this technique (BMJ 1978). Other studies have also supported this range of findings and also added that two-thirds of the detected cancers were confined to the breast and had no evidence of spread. This meant that the survival time of these patients was probably longer than if they had waited for symptoms to appear. It may also have meant less mutilating surgery. Sadly, overall decreased mortality rates are not in evidence.

Routine screening does have certain drawbacks. Many people feel that it encourages more worry by constantly drawing the woman's attention to a disease from which she may not be suffering. Secondly, the woman may end up having unnecessary biopsies to confirm the nonmalignancy of lumps she never knew existed prior to screening. Another danger of screening programmes is the false reassurance given by the yearly check-ups. Women may feel they are protected from one year to the next and will leave their health care with the doctors. In doing so, they may ignore any signs or symptoms which indicate breast disease, and leave them until their next check-up is due.

Many experts also believe that it is unwise to subject the younger age groups to routine annual mammography due to the unknown long term effects of radiation. The general feeling amongst the medical profession appears to be that certain categories of women, that is the 'high risk category', should be screened annually whilst others should be encouraged to perform BSE.

Minimising stress

We must remember that the woman who is undergoing screening procedures because she has found a symptom in her breast may need handling in a different way to the woman who has come for her annual check-up. Firstly, the woman with a symptom has already been through the trauma of its discovery. She may have denied its existence for weeks, months or even years. She may have an accurate idea of what it is, or she may brush aside the implications of it being a cancer. Others may become acutely anxious of their symptom being cancer, and have extinguished all hope of it being anything else Both are coping mechanisms, however good or bad they may seem to us, and it is in adopting such mechanisms that a woman is able to continue her daily chores until the moment of truth arrives.

IN THE DIAGNOSTIC UNIT

So how can we as nurses help minimise the stress caused by these diagnostic techniques? Firstly, a welcoming atmosphere in the diagnostic unit can pave the way in gaining the woman's trust and cooperation. First impressions count and a smile costs nothing! Other nonverbal actions which can help are obvious. Providing adequate privacy is essential, as is adequate heating. Many women are embarrassed by their own nakedness, so it is important that they are not exposed too long before or after examinations. In general, anything that makes women feel more relaxed, such as background music, magazines or access to a cup of coffee, may help to maintain a relaxed atmosphere.

Most women will 'fear the worst'. They tend to forget their friends and acquaintances who have had lumps which have been benign. They tend to forget, or do not know about women they know who have been successfully treated for breast cancer. All they can remember are the friends and relatives who may have died of the disease. These women may be very anxious and difficult to reassure.

PROVIDING INFORMATION

Most women would prefer to know what is happening to them, and results should be given to them in a truthful and tactful manner as soon as they are available. Even so, problems occur for many reasons and the most innocent verbal transaction can take on a new meaning, especially later on in the evening, when the woman starts to reflect on the day's experiences.

One of the common problems is unfamiliar terminology. Such words as glandular, fibrous, nodule, tumour, etc. can sound strange and frightening to many women. You should avoid using such terms when there is insufficient time to explain them, although this can cause some women to feel that there is a 'conspiracy of silence' or they are being 'treated like a child'. To avoid this ask the woman, 'Do you understand what is happening so far?', or 'Is there anything you would like to ask?'; this should give her the opportunity to discuss any worries she may have.

Another problem is that the medical and allied professions seem to use more than one term for certain abnormalities. It would be helpful if there could be a team approach to the terms used, so that the woman does not have a nodule, glandular tissue, tumour or fibrous tissue all in the same visit!

SCREENING FACILITIES

The other side of the coin is seen when women with breast lumps do not undergo screening procedures because there are no facilities available. This may be either a blessing in disguise — no tests, no fear of results, therefore less anxiety, (for the woman and the medical staff) — or this lack of diagnostic tests may leave the woman feeling insecure about her condition and the future management of her disease, should it prove to be cancer.

The media have endeavoured to explain some of the problems of breast lumps and many women question why they are not undergoing these tests. They may not bother to ask the doctor as they may feel he is too busy or unapproachable, but they may ask the nurse. How can she reassure her patient? Firstly, the woman will have a physical examination of both breasts. In experienced hands, the difference between certain abnormalities can be detected: a cyst feels round, skin moves over it easily and fluid can be extracted via a needle. A solid lump is more difficult to diagnose accurately, so a Trucut needle biopsy or aspiration cytology may be performed (Fig. 3.2). Results can be available within a few days, so that the management can be planned. Nipple exudate can also be analysed within a couple of days.

On occasions, these tests may prove inconclusive, but in general they give a fairly accurate picture of whether a malignant or nonmalignant tumour is present. Following one of these procedures the woman may be asked to return to outpatients a week or so later, when the results should be available and treatment can be arranged.

PROVIDING SUPPORT

The waiting period can be quite a difficult time for the woman and her family, as no decisions can be made, and it may seem to her that her future hangs in the balance. Several things can be done to help her over this difficult time.

Firstly, the nurse can ascertain if the woman is emotionally at risk by observing her attitude and listening to what she is saying. If there is a history of breast cancer in her family, and it was one where death occurred, she could be said to be at risk. A woman who has no close friend, be it a partner or relative, could also be at risk, as she may have no-one close enough with whom to talk over her fears and worries. Women with young children may also find difficulty in

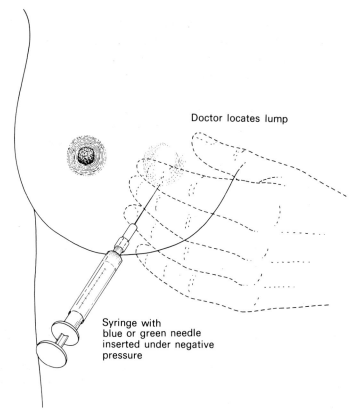

Fig. 3.2   Needle aspiration cytology.

coping if they suspect cancer is present, and of course cancer-phobic people themselves would also need extra help.

By observing those emotionally at risk, the nurse effectively directs her attention to those who need her help, whilst allowing others with adequate coping mechanisms to do so with the minimum of help from the nursing staff until they feel they require it.

Secondly, the nurse can provide a 'lifeline' to the woman. She can do this either by giving the woman the telephone number of the unit and the name of someone to talk to (herself or Sister), should the need arise, or she can refer her to the appropriate health visitor, giving a brief outline of what is happening. If there are identifiable social problems such as financial or marital worries, then the social worker, with the woman's permission, may also be called upon. In other words, taking the whole woman and not just her breast lump into consideration means better care, better understanding and a smoother course for both the patient and the team of people who will eventually be looking after her.

There should be no need to emphasise that the woman is the *leader* of this team, and makes her decisions with our help. If she is encouraged to be actively involved from the time she is diagnosed, then she will feel in control of the course of events.

Trucut biopsy

The role of the nurse is firstly to assist her patient through the procedure of a Trucut biopsy, and secondly to aid the doctor to ensure the smooth running and efficiency of the test.

Problem.   The patient needs to know what is going to happen and why.
Action.   Give a simple explanation, e.g. the skin over the lump will be cleansed and a small needle will be used to inject a local anaesthetic. When the the skin is numb, a sample of tissue will be taken by inserting a larger needle into the lump. This will be sent to the laboratory so that it can be analysed.

Problem.   The patient's fear of the unknown.
Action.   Although the immediate procedure has been explained, she needs to be reassured about the nature of her disease. Tell her that the results will be available when she comes back next week (*see* Chapter 7).

Problem.   The patient needs to be aware of what is the next stage.
Action.   The patient needs to be informed that once home, the dressing will be able to come off when she has a bath. In addition, 'We would like you to come back next week to this department to see Mr Jones, we will have the results by then. Will you be coming alone or would you like to bring your partner/sister?' or similar information needs to given.

EXERCISE

Let us return to Katherine, the patient we discussed at the end of Chapter 2. After she has undergone investigations in the outpatient department, the surgeon decides that the lump in Katherine's left breast is 'suspicious' and arranges for her to be admitted to hospital to have the lump excised under general anaesthetic.

1 As the nurse in the outpatient department, how could you prepare Katherine for this forthcoming admission to hospital?
2 You read in Katherine's medical notes that the surgeon has staged the lump in her breast as follows:

T 1a, N 1b, M 0

What exactly does this mean?

REFERENCES

BMJ (1978) Screening for Breast Cancer: Report from the Edinburgh Breast Screening Clinic. *British Medical Journal* **2**, 175-8.

Bovee, W.M.M.J. & Getreuer, K.W., (1978) Nuclear magnetic resonance and detection of human breast tumours. *Journal of the National Cancer Institute* **61**, 53-5.

Moskowitz M., Milbrath, J. & Gartside, P. (1976) Lack of efficacy of thermography as a screening tool for minimal and stage 1 breast cancer. *New England Journal of Medicine* **295**, 249-52.

FURTHER READING

British Breast Group. (1978) Screening for Breast Cancer. Statement by British Breast Group. *British Medical Journal* **2**, 178-80.

Burger, D. (1979) Breast Self-Examination. *American Journal of Nursing* **79**(6), 1088-9.

Burger, D. (1979) A Plain Woman's Guide to BSE (Self-Examination). Community Outlook, *Nursing Times* **75**, 312-13.

Davey, J. (1978) Screening, The Pre-symptomatic Diagnosis of Cancer. In *Oncology for Nurses and Health Care Professionals*, R. Tiffany (ed.). Allen & Unwin, London.

Edinburgh Breast Screening Clinic (1978) Screening for Breast Cancer. Report from the Screening Clinic. *British Medical Journal* **2**, 175-8.

Edwards, V. (1980) Changing Breast Self-Examination Behaviour. *Nursing Res.* **29**(5) 301-6.

Hobbs, P. *et al.* (1977) Motivation and Education in Breast Cancer Screening. (Review of Recent Studies.) *Public Health* **91**(5), 249-52.

Hobbs, P. *et al.* (1980) Acceptors and Rejectors of an Invitation to Undergo Breast Screening Compared with those who Referred Themselves. *Journal of Epidemiol/Community Health* **34** (1), 19–22.

Howe, H.L. (1980) Proficiency in Performing Breast Self-Examination. (Tests on Silicone models showing more instruction is needed.) *Pat. Couns. Health Education* **2** (4), 151-7.

Hubbard, S.M. (1978) Breast Cancer: Nurse's Role is Vital In Early Detection. (Risk factors, screening procedures, diagnosis and treatments.) *Nursing Mirror* **147**, 31-7.

Smith, T. (1981) *Early Detection. Breast Cancer.* Gerald Duckworth, London.

Stillman, M.J. (1977) Women's Health Beliefs about Breast Cancer and Breast Self-Examination. *Nursing Res.* **26**(2), 121-7.

Chapter 4
Surgery as Primary Treatment

Because surgery is seen as a primary means of treatment for breast cancer, the nurse's relationship to patients undergoing surgery becomes a first line of treatment. Specific nursing care is presented in terms of identifying patient nursing problems and potential problems and outlining possible nursing actions which could be taken to solve or prevent problems. Let us, therefore, explore:

1 Types of operation which are considered as a means of primary surgical intervention for breast cancer.

2 Related patient problems arising from each surgical procedure and nursing actions which might alleviate these.

3 Factors which should contribute to a decision as to which surgical procedure is most appropriate to each individual patient.

HISTORICAL PERSPECTIVE

Historically, breast cancer was defined as a local disease and, as such, surgical intervention was aimed at removing all possible cancer cells in the breast. Mastectomy of varying types and degrees has been performed on women since the ancient Greek and Roman times. In the 1700s and 1800s surgeons were advocating removal of axillary lymph nodes as well. One such surgeon, Symes, whose advice has largely been ignored until recent years, suggested in 1842 that, if the breast cancer had spread to the lymph glands at the time of operation, it probably indicated that it also had spread to other parts of the body.

In 1890, Halsted described a new radical mastectomy which he was carrying out. This involved removing the entire breast along with the pectoralis major and pectoralis minor muscles and all the axillary lymph glands. This extensive operation remains the conventional and standard surgical procedure in most parts of the world today.

34

Even more extensive surgery has been advocated by surgeons in the past and is termed an extended or supraradical mastectomy. This involves lifting a flap of tissue from the chest wall at the time of operation to remove the lymph nodes in the internal mammary chain (*see* Fig. 1.1 showing lymph glands surrounding the breast). In some cases, ribs in the affected area have also been removed.

These radical procedures were considered the best course of action for primary surgical treatment of breast cancer for several reasons:

1   As noted, breast cancer was always believed to be a local disease.
2   The aim of surgery was clearly defined and understood — to remove surgically all breast tissue, surrounding muscle and lymph glands in order to effect a cure.
3   Staging procedures and their implications were largely unknown and poorly understood.
4   The nature of breast cancer was poorly understood.

Recent changes

In recent years clinical trials have been carried out under carefully monitored conditions to see if other surgical procedures could alter the long-term survival rate of women with breast cancer. At the same time, new advances in staging breast cancer have come to light (*see* Chapter 2) as well as new understanding of the nature of breast cancer. What seems to be evident is that no one surgical procedure has demonstrated that it produces a better long-term survival rate than any other surgical procedure. It does appear that radical mastectomy may prevent local recurrence of breast cancer at the site of operation. It has been reconfirmed what Symes discovered in 1842 — that axillary node involvement at the time of operation is an indicator of the disease possibly having spread elsewhere. This means that presence of tumour spread to the axilla probably indicates metastases or micrometastases elsewhere. Because of this, the objectives of surgery as primary treatment have changed considerably.

These recent discoveries about breast cancer are important to nurses. Nurses need to establish good communication with medical staff as to the objectives of any surgery which is being planned. This shift in thinking about surgery for breast cancer also indicates a change in the thinking of surgeons who once believed that 'all patients with breast cancer must have a radical mastectomy'. Surgeons must now view each patient and the prospective surgery they might undertake in terms of the stage of the disease, the objective of surgery for each patient, and the age of the patient — with particular reference to the patient's ability to cope psychologically with the end results of surgery.

The modern *objectives* of surgery when deciding the appropriate primary treatment for women with breast cancer are:

1   Full clinical staging must be carried out prior to deciding which surgical procedure is most appropriate.

2   After staging, all possible surgical alternatives are considered.

3   In some cases, the decision as to which surgical procedure is most appropriate may involve considering what adjuvant treatment might be necessry postoperatively, (e.g. radiotherapy or chemotherapy).

4   Even if 'cure' is not feasible because of known metastatic spread, surgery might be indicated to alleviate or prevent local spread of the disease, such as ulceration. Here, surgery is used as primary treatment to achieve a better quality of life.

Surgical treatment

AS A CURE

Surgeons who advocated mastectomy with total removal of axillary glands are gradually realising that radical and extended radical mastectomy can be replaced by less drastic, less mutilating surgery which can achieve the same desired end result.

The *modified radical mastectomy* is one such operation. This procedure involves removal of the breast, division of the pectoralis minor muscle and removal of axillary glands. The pectoralis major is left intact. This operation is less disfiguring in that it is far easier for the woman to regain symmetry with breast prostheses than was possible with more radical surgery. A greater variety of low neckline clothing can be worn without it being obvious that the woman has undergone breast surgery.

Some surgeons are now becoming more concerned with Symes' findings and are realising that, if there is lymph node involvement at the time of diagnosis, then there probably is microscopic systemic metastases. For this reason many surgeons now believe that even a modified radical mastectomy is inappropriate. These surgeons are moving to a surgical procedure which involves a wide excision of the tumour (removal of tumour and several centimetres of normal tissue surrounding the tumour) with axillary clearance (removal of the lower two-thirds of the axillary chain of glands). This is usually followed by a course of radiotherapy to the breast and axilla and sometimes will include a course of prophylactic chemotherapy as additional adjuvant treatment.

In women who have been diagnosed as having carcinoma in situ or premalignant conditions such as Paget's disease of the nipple, simple mastectomy is the operation of choice. This involves removal only of the breast; all the muscles and local lymph glands are retained.

TREATING OR PREVENTING LOCAL RECURRENCE

Many surgeons have chosen to perform radical mastectomy in an attempt to prevent local recurrence of the disease. Recently, however, surgeons have been trying to begin with more conservative surgical intervention to minimise postoperative complications and disfigurement of the woman. Either way, there are obvious dilemmas present in deciding upon the most appropriate choice of surgery and there is a great need for priorities of surgery and treatment to be well thought out.

Baum (1981) points out that the most important thing for surgeons to remember is that, in the absence of long-term clinical evidence indicating that one approach is better than another, no surgeon should have fixed, inflexible ideas about surgical treatment of women with breast cancer. Nurses too should be aware that there is little evidence to indicate that one type of operation is any better than any other.

DETERMINING APPROPRIATE INTERVENTION

In Chapter 2 we outlined the basis of the clinical staging of breast cancer. This staging must play a large part in the decision as to the most appropriate surgical intervention in each patient. For this reason, nurses should be aware of the staging of their patients with breast cancer in order both to be able to give informed answers to questions about possible treatment which might be asked by patients and relatives, and also to reinforce and iterate explanations given by medical staff.

Extent of metastatic spread (if any) at the time of presentation of the patient can only be ascertained through various scanning procedures such as liver scan and bone scan. These are discussed in greater depth in Chapter 12. If metastatic disease is already present it is pointless to subject a woman to a mutilating procedure such as a mastectomy. Mastectomy, regardless of type preferred by the surgeon, must only be used if the aim is cure or if there is a high risk of fungating lesion or local recurrence. If clinical staging is carried out preoperatively and metastases are found to be present, the aim of surgery is *not* for cure but for removal of as much of the tumour as possible prior to other forms of treatment such as adjuvant radiotherapy, chemotherapy or hormone therapy. Regardless of what surgery is to be performed staging must be carried out first on all patients with breast cancer.

Size of tumour might also play a part in determining the type of surgical procedure chosen. If the tumour is a large one (e.g. greater than 5 cm), a wide excision might be less desirable because the amount of tissue which would need to be removed might make it difficult for the woman to regain symmetry postoperatively. In this case, regardless of absence or presence of metastases, a mastectomy might be the most appropriate operation for cosmetic reasons.

Fungation of the skin over the tumour will affect decisions about the most appropriate surgical procedure for a woman with breast cancer. Usually, the skin overlying the breast is used to cover the chest wall after the breast tissue has been removed. But if the skin has fungated, it means that the cancer has spread to this skin making it impossible for it to be retained. In these cases attempts have been made to use means of grafting skin and other appropriate tissue to cover the breast site after mastectomy and removal of the fungating lesion. Two such surgical techniques which are carried out for fungating breast lesions are omentum swings and latissimus dorsi. These are only carried out in specialist centres and are therefore not procedures with which many nurses will need to be familiar.

Age is another consideration which must be taken into account when a decision about surgery is being made. Younger women who present with breast cancer may not be able to cope with the thought of a mutilating breast operation. Those who present with tumours which are small and have been diagnosed early may be considered for subcutaneous mastectomy with a silicone implant. This operation is described in greater depth in Chapter 5. Psychological factors must also be considered with a careful assessment of the patient's ability to cope and adjust to mastectomy. Many hospitals are beginning to see the importance of this and are employing specialist mastectomy nurses to counsel patients before and after surgery to assess their ability to cope and come to terms with their illness. The role of specialist nurses in this field is detailed by two such nurses in Chapters 7 and 8.

Regardless of the facts available and the surgeon's own decision about the most appropriate surgical procedure, the wishes and desires of the woman herself and those of her husband/partner in life must also be considered. This is where the subject of *informed consent* becomes so important. The patient must be given enough accurate information about her disease and possible outcome to make an informed decision about surgery and treatment. The role of the nurse is to be informed herself so she can reinforce the information given by the surgeon and so that she can support the patient in whatever decision she makes.

NURSING MANAGEMENT FOR PATIENTS UNDERGOING PRIMARY SURGERY

The nursing management for patients involves identifying patients' problems or possible problems and determining nursing actions to either manage or prevent these problems. Each type of operation can lead to different actual or possible nursing problems for the woman by the very nature of the amount of tissue which is being removed and long- and short-term implications of the operation. For this reason, this section of the chapter on nursing management is divided into two parts: nursing management following a simple mastectomy, and nursing management following more extensive surgery (wide excision with axillary clearance, modified radical and radical mastectomy).

Simple mastectomy

The long term goals or aims of care are:
— clean wound
— patient feels pain free
— patient understands operation
— patient is able to carry out usual activities of daily living.

Problem.   Anxiety due to surgery, fear of diagnosis and unfamiliar surroundings.
Action.   Explain hospital routines and surroundings.
Preoperative teaching about operation and what to expect postoperatively (amount of pain, how nurses will aid its control, dressings and bandages, arm position, intravenous infusion, etc. *see* Hayward, 1974.)

Problem.   Pain due to surgery, possible haematoma or postoperative fluid collection under suture line, or from anxiety.
Action.   Good, comfortable arm positioning postoperatively with arm elevated on a pillow(s).
Encourage deep breathing exercises to relax and relieve muscle tightness.
Offer analgesia as prescribed and evaluate by asking the patient about its effectiveness after half an hour and again after two or three hours.

Problem.   Possible wound infection due to fluid collection beneath suture line or due to haematoma.

Action.   Check vacuum drains two-hourly.

Measure and record drainage daily or more frequently if required.

Daily temperature recordings.

Daily observation of wound or dressing for blood loss, tenderness, redness, swelling and pain. Re-dress as required using aseptic technique.

Problem.   Possible depression/anxiety/fear of rejection due to altered body image.

Action.   Stay with patient after first dressing change. Allow her as much time as she needs to talk about her fear.

Do not force her to look at suture line until she feels ready. But she should be encouraged to do so before discharge.

Teach her about the work of the Mastectomy Association and when appropriate, give her one of their booklets to read.

Continually help her to express her feelings and help her to maintain a realistic outlook.

If appropriate, encourage husband/partner to look at mastectomy site whilst patient is still in hospital.

Problem.   Embarrassment and possible feelings of withdrawal due to fear of looking abnormal.

Action.   Fit temporary prosthesis ('comfy' or 'cosy') as soon as she is pain free or when sutures are removed.

Arrange with mastectomy nurse specialist or fitter for permanent prosthesis to be supplied.

Advise about bras and clothing (*see* Chapter 6).

Problem.   Fear about possible future treatment and prognosis.

Action.   Reinforce and re-explain information from medical staff, if appropriate.

Give accurate factual information about any future treatment, possible side-effects, etc. in language which the patient can understand.

If patient is to have follow-up radiotherapy, take her to the radiotherapy department to see the machines and meet the radiographer.

OTHER NURSING CARE

It has not been the intention of this chapter to include some of the more basic aspects of nursing care. For example, one of the goals of nursing care for patients undergoing simple mastectomy is the ability to carry out activities of daily living. Those activities of living basic to the woman (such as hygiene) would have been carried out by the nurse when the patient was too ill to do so by herself but, upon discharge, the patient would be caring for her own activities of living unaided. As well as the problems (or possible problems) mentioned in the care plan for a patient undergoing simple mastectomy, any other problems for this woman would have been identified on admission with a good nursing history or some other sort of organised information gathering. For these individually identified problems, suitable nursing actions would also have to be planned and care given and evaluated accordingly.

Extensive surgery

Patients who undergo extensive surgery involving wide excision with axillary dissection, modified radical and radical mastectomy will have the same long range aims or goals as discussed previously for patients undergoing simple mastectomy. In addition, they will have another goal: to be able to move their arm fully. The problem-orientated nursing care for these patients will include many of the problems and possible problems as for patients undergoing simple mastectomy and many of the same nursing actions. For example, where a patient, who has undergone simple mastectomy, is concerned at looking abnormal the fitting of temporary and permanent prostheses is recommended above. For patients undergoing wide excision, however, the need would be for a partial prosthesis. These are not always easy to obtain or to fit. The advice on bras and clothing would also be slightly different for this latter group and this, too, will be discussed in Chapter 7.

In addition to the problems identified for patients undergoing simple mastectomy, the following are problems or possible problems which will need to be considered for those undergoing a wide excision with axillary dissection (or axillary clearance), modified radical or radical mastectomy.

Problem. Possible lymphoedema due to surgical removal of axillary glands.
Action. Elevate arm postoperatively until mobilising.
Nurse to use patient's unaffected arm for taking blood pressure. Blood samples should also be taken from the unaffected side.
See Chapter 12 for complete care and prevention of lymphoedema.

Problem. Possible limited arm movements due to axillary surgery.
Action. Refer to physiotherapist for arm exercises. Encourage patient to carry out exercises as prescribed by physiotherapist. This is often useful to do as a group with all patients doing exercises together. Encourage patient to carry out those activities which specifically use raised arm movements, such as combing hair and brushing teeth.

As with the care plan for simple mastectomy, the above problems, possible problems and related nursing actions include only care which is specific to the problems which arise or might possibly arise from the operations. Basic nursing care is omitted and again the emphasis must be on finding out the patients' usual pattern of daily living activities, social history and other information in order to plan and give total individualised care. The use of long-term goals — or goals for discharge — is a good way of ensuring that all nurses are aiming for the same end result in their care of the patient and that progress can be monitored on the basis of these goals.

EXERCISE

Katherine and her husband are seen by the surgeon who explains the results of the biopsy report after the excision of the lump. The report shows that the lump is an infiltrating intraduct adenocarcinoma. The surgeon advises that Katherine undergo modified radical mastectomy.
1 How would you explain this operation to Katherine and her husband? Would your explanation be different if you were explaining it to a junior nurse on your ward rather than to the patient?

2   Discuss ways in which the nursing staff might help Katherine and her husband during this difficult time.

3   Using a problem-solving approach write a plan of care for Katherine's postoperative period. Remember to identify actual or possible problems she might encounter. Think about the aims of the nursing care you might give. What care would you give and how would you evaluate the progress of each problem?

REFERENCES

Baum, M. (1981) *Breast Cancer: The Facts.* Oxford University Press.
Hayward, J. (1974) *Information — A Prescription Against Pain.* Rcn, London.

Chapter 5
Breast Reconstruction

There is an old adage that says 'It is better to be flat chested and alive rather than a good-looking corpse'. However, whilst there is no doubt that many women who have had mastectomies have come to terms with their altered body image and external prostheses, others have great difficulty in coping with their disfigurements. If we examine what has happened in the medical world over the past few years, we may be able to find out why attitudes are changing.

The media have in recent years devoted more and more time to medical topics, with the aim of educating the public about their bodies. Breast cancer has naturally been included in this type of coverage, so that more women and their families are aware of the various possibilities of treatment, including breast reconstruction. Many years ago, plastic surgery was a luxury only the very rich could afford. Nowadays, we are seeing an increasing amount of plastic surgery being performed under the NHS, as doctors are realising that their duty should be to restore the patient to wholeness, both physically and psychologically, as well as ridding them of their disease.

Other factors which have made breast reconstruction more feasible are that surgical techniques have changed over the years, leading to less radical surgery being performed. The cosmetic results of implant surgery have been greatly improved, so that plastic surgeons are able to convince their fellow surgeons that it can be a worthwhile procedure (Fig. 5.1).

The question of how long a woman should have to wait before undergoing reconstructive surgery is not clear, and surgeons are divided on the issue. Some feel that implants should be performed at the time of initial surgery, as they say there is little point in waiting. They feel the woman has a better chance of psychological recovery if

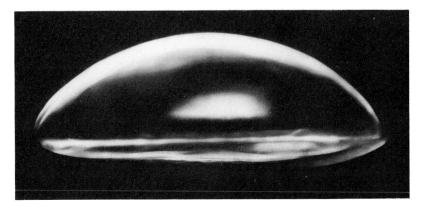

Fig. 5.1 A silastic mammary implant. The thick envelope makes the implant more resistant to rupture. It is made from 100% medical graded silicone materials and is essentially non-reactive to body tissue. (Photography courtesy of Dow Corning.)

she does not 'lose' the breast at all. This type of implant — subcutaneous mastectomy — would seem feasible for a very small non-invasive tumour such as carcinoma in situ because the risk of not being able to remove all the tumour is very small and the overall prognosis good. A problem arises in that two surgeons, the plastic surgeon and cancer surgeon both have to be present at the operation. However in certain hospitals there may be a surgeon who is expert in both fields. Other doctors feel that the ideal time is anywhere between three months and three years post mastectomy. The large variation in time is accounted for by the surgeon's feelings about local recurrence and breast cancer itself and the amount of time needed for the skin and underlying tissue to heal.

Who?

So who is eligible for implant surgery? First, age is no barrier; all that is required is that the patient is fit enough to undergo a general anaesthetic. Patients who have had previous skin grafts or radiotherapy to the chest may not be entirely suitable candidates as their skin may not stretch enough to accommodate the implant, but each patient must be assessed on an individual basis. Women who have had radical surgery may lack skin and pectoral muscle to accommodate the implant and usually need extensive surgery to fill in the chest and axilla.

Why?

The next point we must look at are the reasons for the woman requesting reconstructive surgery. Some of the reasons given for wanting an implant have been divided into practical/social and psychological categories.

PRACTICAL/SOCIAL

My clothes don't look right. (A common problem if a radical operation has been performed.)

I would feel better if I didn't have to wear a prosthesis when swimming and playing other sports.

I can't wear plunging necklines which show a cleavage.

I would like to wear low-cut 'flimsy' bras and bikinis.

I am not happy wearing an external prosthesis.

I want to feel I have two breasts like any other woman.

PSYCHOLOGICAL

My relationship with my husband/partner is unstable and I think an implant would improve this.

I feel I have lost part of my sexual attractiveness and identity.

My self-esteem has been lowered since my mastectomy.

I feel I have not fully accepted the mastectomy and an implant would help.

The mastectomy scar and loss of breast is a constant reminder that I have had a disease.

The first group of patients' problems can be rectified in most cases by an implant. These are women who want practical solutions to their practical problems. For the second group however, an implant alone will not solve their problems, although it may go a long way towards helping them achieve their goal. They will also need help from a counsellor or psychotherapist so that the underlying emotional problems can be dealt with.

Possible complications of breast implants

There are, however, some drawbacks to the surgery, and the wise surgeon will point these out to the patient. They are listed below:
1   Infection of the wound may occur postoperatively.
2   Capsule formation is a possible risk.
3   The body may reject the implant, though this is an extremely rare complication.
4   The bosom will not look like or match the natural breast.
5   The other breast may need surgery in order to achieve a more balanced look, e.g. a 'droopy' bosom may need a surgical uplift, whilst a large bosom may need a reduction mammoplasty.

Often the patient turns to the nurse to discuss these side-effects, so we can look at them in a little more detail.

Infection may be a problem in the postoperative period, though it is usually successfully treated by administering the appropriate systemic antibiotic. Should wound breakdown occur, the surgeon may have to remove the implant until the skin has completely healed.

Capsule formation occurs in a percentage of women, and is characterised by excessive breast firmness and discomfort. It is thought that firm, daily massage of the breast and implant commencing 4–6 weeks after surgery may either prevent or delay the onset of this reaction. Should a fibrous capsule form, it can be relieved by external manipulation which is often done in the outpatient department, either with or without a short general anaesthetic. Sometimes the only option is to cut the fibrous capsule around the implant, which will necessitate an overnight stay in hospital.

The fact that the implant will not exactly match the remaining breast should be pointed out prior to surgery, as the woman will be very disappointed if she expected a perfect replica. The whole idea of an implant is that it should look good in a bra, a cleavage should be evident, and there is no need to wear a prosthesis of any kind. If these criteria have been fulfilled, the operation may be considered a success.

Care of the preoperative patient entails ensuring she is fully aware of the possible outcome of surgery. She will need to have a comfortable, well-fitting bra before surgery (*see* Chapter 3). Sports bras are not suitable for the postoperative period because, althought they have the right type of support, they generally have an elasticated top, which would dig in to the oedematous implanted breast. Some surgeons require their patients to wear specialised bras which have moulded cups in them, in order to keep the implant in place, whilst others are happy with an ordinary bra providing it fits properly. Sometimes the bra accompanies the patient to the operating theatre and is put on immediately after surgery.

The axilla should be shaved prior to surgery, but apart from this there are no other specific nursing preparations.

Care of the postoperative patient largely depends upon the surgeon's wishes, as techniques at present are so varied. If drainage of the wound is necessary, these will remain in for the first 24 hours and removed when drainage is minimal. Sutures are usually left in situ for 14 days — longer if the patient has previously had radiotherapy to the chest. Arm movements are generally restricted in the first three weeks. The patient must be instructed not to elevate her arm above shoulder level for this period. Full arm movements may be gradually increased after this period.

The patient is usually discharged 4–5 days postoperatively and is followed-up in the plastic surgeon's clinic to ensure that the implant has been successful. The outpatient nurse will be in a position to instruct her patient on how to massage the implanted breast which will help to stop capsule formation.

EXERCISE

Prior to surgery, Katherine's surgeon had discussed with her the possibility of breast reconstruction in the future. Katherine and her husband decided to think about this option and discuss it with each other.

1   What are the advantages and disadvantages of Katherine having this breast reconstruction?

FURTHER READING

Miller S.H. *et al.* (1977) Breast Reconstruction Following Mastectomy. (An Implantable Silicone Prosthesis). *AORN J* **25**(5), 945, 948-9.

Gray, S. (1981) International Cancer Nursing Conference 10. Breast Restoration. (Recent Changes in Treatment) *Nursing Mirror* **152**, 40-2.

McDowell, P.G. & Wylie, M.E. (1980) Mastectomy and Insertion of Prosthesis. (Details of Operation and Review of Psychological Aspects). *Nursing Times* **76**, 1258-61.

Chapter 6
Prostheses and Clothing

'Three tenths of a woman's good looks are due to nature, seven tenths to dress' (ancient Chinese proverb).

BRAS — YESTERDAY AND TODAY

Bra is a diminutive form of the word brassière and the origins of the word are now lost. The Greeks probably invented the first bra or breast band — the mastodeton — and the aim was probably to flatten the breasts. During the 16th Century, whale bone corsets and bodices were used to encase women into the prevailing fashion, whilst the Regency fashion of the 1800s led to an invention known as bust improvers or false bosoms, quaintly known as 'bosom friends'. Victorian busts were well supported and matronly in appearance, and it is thought that these undergarments were nearer to the idea of modern supports than many of the previous eras of fashion. Edwardian ladies preferred beauty and lace to the more commonsense attitude of their Victorian mothers, though shapes remained unnaturally restricting and fashion conscious.

It was not until the 1920s that the bra became the garment that we know today. Ideas of restriction and flattening, enhancing and enlarging went by the wayside and gave rise to a garment which followed the natural contours and weight of the breast. After extensive analysis on thousands of women, both Berli and Warner Brothers came up with sizing which meant a woman could buy a ready-made bra to suit her. The idea of bra fittings being as easy as ABC had emerged. Pointed conical breasts were all the fashion and a whole industry had been born to cater for those whom nature had underendowed. As women became more liberated and started to dictate fashion themselves, so the fashion of bras changed.

Today it is estimated that in the UK we spend nearly £150 million each year on bras. Women choose bras to wear for comfort, though many 'fun' and leisure bras are bought for social reasons. Many women do not have the correct fitting bra, either because they do not realise they have the wrong style and size, or because they are too embarrassed to be fitted professionally. As nurses we may be required to give some general advice on the right type of bra to wear postoperatively, whether or not the patient has had her breast removed. Below are listed a few general hints on how to check that your patient is wearing the right kind of bra.

1 The bra should not cause any red marks to appear on the skin. Strap marks occur if the breasts are not adequately supported, or if the straps have been pulled too high.

2 The breasts should not be able to move about inside the bra cup; this is caused by a bra which is too loose around the rib cage or has too large a cup size.

3 The breast should be completely encased in the cup. If excess breast tissue is allowed to 'spill out' then the cup size needs to be larger.

4 The bra should feel comfortable.

5 Wired bras are not really suitable for postoperative wear.

If the patient's bra gives rise to any of these problems, the nurse should advise her to visit a suitable shop or department store which will be able to supply her with a correctly fitting bra. It may also be necessary to inform patients that the requirements for support to the breasts change as the years pass by, so that a 20-year-old woman wearing a 36B will need a different kind of support from a 65-year-old 36B. The fact that the woman may not have gained any weight during her life-time does not mean that she will always need the same size or style of bra.

It is curious to note that over the past 5–10 years, the average British woman's bust size has increased from a 34B to a 36C. Could better nutrition, the 'Pill' and exercise be underlying factors?

Post mastectomy

The nurse is in a unique position to offer practical advice because she is often the person who has the most clinical contact with her patient. She should therefore be able to encourage her patient to discuss any potential problems associated with regaining symmetry and have the knowledge and expertise to advise her accordingly.

The patient's psychological adjustment depends on many factors as we will see in Chapters 7 and 8, but providing adequate practical advice about prostheses, bras, swimwear and clothing will be of enormous help and encouragement to her.

Nightwear/hospital wear

As many mastectomies are performed within a few weeks of the woman visiting her GP, she may not have given much thought to the kind of hospital nightdresses which would be suitable for postoperative wear. It is essential for her mental well-being that postoperatively she feels presentable for visitors and other patients on the ward. A lack of a breast can be quite disconcerting for a large-breasted woman, and she should be offered a temporary prosthesis within the first few days of her operation, which she can secure into her nightdress. A smaller breasted woman may be able to by-pass this stage by wearing a loosely fitting or yoked nightdress (Fig. 6.1). Whichever approach is adopted, it should be handled with care and sensitivity. Addresses for suitable types of temporary prostheses can be found in Appendix 3.

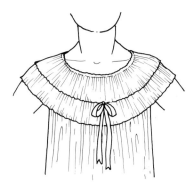

Fig. 6.1 A yoked nightdress.

Going home — fitting a temporary prosthesis

A woman's first steps out of hospital are immensely important and every effort should be made by the nursing staff to ensure that she looks exactly as she did when she entered hospital. She should be asked to wear an outfit that is not too tight, but at the same time is attractive and flatters her figure. It should be emphasised that the temporary prosthesis is for the first few postoperative weeks only and that a more permanent prosthesis will be fitted around 6–8 weeks.

Fitting a temporary prosthesis requires skill and sensitivity. They are available in sizes AA to D and in most types the Dacron wool filling can be supplemented or removed as required. It is also important to ensure that the contours at the side of the 'bosom' are not neglected, so that some wool will have to be rearranged into the axillary area. Because of the difference in weight between the temporary prosthesis and the remaining breast the bra straps may have to be adjusted — higher on the side of the remaining breast and lower on the mastectomy side. In teaching the woman how to fit her temporary prosthesis one must remember that the wool will need repositioning each time she wears a different type of bra, or after washing the breast form. If her skin is still very sensitive and she does not feel able to wear her bra, she need not go home looking lop-sided as the temporary prosthesis may be worn tucked inside her petticoat and secured with a safety pin or press stud. Before she goes home she should be offered information on the choice of permanent breast forms and told how to get in touch with the appropriate fitting department.

Fitting the right prosthesis is essential if a woman is to regain her confidence and pick up the threads of her life. The optimum time for fitting the permanent prosthesis is approximately 6–8 weeks postoperatively, as fitting before she leaves hospital, during radiotherapy or before the wound has sufficiently healed will only lead to an incorrect fit.

As we have seen, the right type of bra is one that has a good support and covers all of the remaining breast tissue. Whilst one endeavours to fit the prosthesis into the type of bra the women wore preoperatively, the problems of doing so if the bra is not suitable must be pointed out, as a comfortable fitting cannot be guaranteed. However, one must take into account that the woman may not be able to afford a new bra. Also, she may require a larger-sized bra which, after fitting the prosthesis, may mean her clothes would no longer fit around the bust.

If fitted correctly the prosthesis should not need securing into position. However, many women feel insecure and prefer to sew a pocket into the back of the bra, enabling the prosthesis to be slipped in. Pocketing is also available through the NHS at no cost to the patient. (The cost to the hospital is approximately £3–4 per pocket.) A simpler way of securing the prosthesis in place is that of criss-cross tapes (Fig. 6.2). This is a relatively simple task which can be done by the woman herself using either bias binding or baby ribbon. An alternative is to buy a specially made mastectomy bra through retail outlets (*see* Appendix 3).

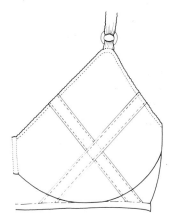

Fig. 6.2   Criss-cross tapes sewn inside the cup of an ordinary bra.

Many women who have undergone mastectomy have said that their prosthesis, and the way in which it was fitted, gave rise to a great deal of dissatisfaction. Indeed, in a study by Downie in 1974, it was shown that 42% of women were not satisfied with their artificial bosoms. This problem should not occur nowadays, as there are many prostheses available under the NHS. There is no such thing as a 'bad' prosthesis, all have their good points, and whilst one woman will find one particular type suitable for her, another woman will not. It is extremely important therefore that the woman should be able to choose her false bosom from the full range available.

The Aysmoena silicone prosthesis (Fig. 6.3a) is suitable for a 'simple mastectomy'. Note the round shape. It is available in nine sizes, can be worn on either the left or right side, is easy to wash, and comes supplied with covers. An elliptical shaped prosthesis (Fig. 6.3b) is also available, in ten sizes, and is suitable for women who have lost axillary tissue. The Amoena silicone breastform (Fig. 6.3c) is designed for use on either the left or right side. It is available in twelve sizes and comes supplied with covers. The Amoena heart-shaped silicone prosthesis (Fig. 6.3d) can be worn in three different positions to compensate for loss of pectoral or axillary tissue. It is available in nine sizes.

The DHSS policy on supplying and resupplying false bosoms is quite specific, and enables the woman to have the right to choose whichever bosom she wishes. It also ensures that she is supplied with a false breast when hers is worn, and states that it should always be a replica of the remaining bosom.

The fitting

The first fitting of a breast prosthesis is extremely important. These are points to remember on your patient's behalf.

1   The woman has the right to request that she be fitted by a female fitter.

2   Fittings are not done by bra sizes. As we have seen, many women are not wearing the correct bra size anyway, so that fitting her with a size 3 of any style because size 3 is supposed to fit a 36B will be of no use if her correct size is 38C.

3   A friend/husband should be encouraged to accompany her for this fitting, as they can often cast a more critical eye over the finished shape than she can and give helpful advice if needed.

4   The woman should have a choice of *all* the types available, and should not be limited to one or two styles.

5   She should be shown how to insert the prosthesis correctly, and how to take care of it.

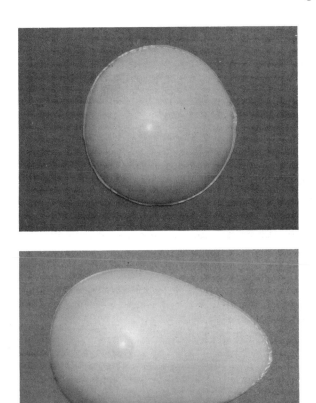

Fig. 6.3   Different types and shapes of prosthesis available (a–d; *see also overleaf*). (Photographs courtesy of Camp Ltd.)

6   She should be told how long the prosthesis is expected to last and how to apply for a new false bosom. But she should also be informed that if she gains or loses weight, she can apply for a new one.

If these guidelines are followed, a successful fitting should be the result, and no-one should be able to see or feel the difference. Whilst one realises that financial constraints limit many hospitals with regard to the range of fittings, and indeed the fitting rooms themselves, it does not help the patient's morale to be told of the cost

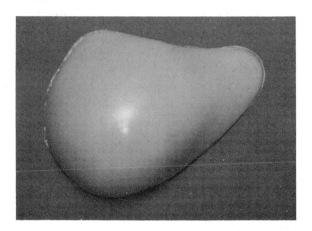

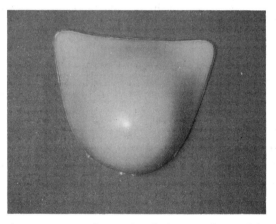

of her false bosom, or to have the fitting performed in a cramped office cluttered with wheelchairs and false limbs.

An ideal room is one that has adequate natural lighting, a full length mirror and possibly a couple of easy chairs, so that the whole procedure can be undertaken in a relaxed atmosphere. This may be the first time the woman has actually confronted her own body since her operation, therefore the fitting should be handled in a sensitive manner. For an expert fitter, finding the 'right bosom' will take no longer than 10–15 minutes, but she will also realise that this is too short a time for the woman to choose such an intimate part of her apparel, and will give her a little more time to choose, perhaps by leaving her alone to browse and try them on in privacy.

Another point on which most good fitters would agree is that it is no good fitting the prosthesis into the bra whilst the woman is standing upright like a tin soldier! She needs to perform some of her daily activities such as reaching up to cupboards, bending and stretching. If any problems come to light then either the prosthesis or bra is unsuitable; alternatively if it is just one particular activity such as bending which is giving rise to problems, pocketing may be advisable.

THE NURSE'S ROLE

What is the nurse's role in prosthetics and fittings? We have seen how her role should cover fitting the first temporary prosthesis whilst the patient is in hospital (Chapter 6). It is also her duty to ensure that the patient knows how and when to get in touch with the surgical appliance department — perhaps the fitter's name and telephone extension number, together with an appointment, may be helpful.

The nurse in the outpatients department has a special part to play as the patient may be too nervous about her follow-up visit to remember to ask about a new bosom when hers no longer fits or has worn. The nurse can enquire about this directly, so that it becomes a nurse-to-patient (and woman-to-woman) transaction, rather than a patient-to-doctor request, as patients dislike asking doctors to fill out yet another form.

FOLLOW-UP

Many patients are only followed-up for five years after a mastectomy and then discharged to the care of their GP, but their need for a false bosom will continue for the rest of their lives. A patient should be aware that she can get a request form from her GP which will be sent to her local hospital for her fitting. At no time should she be made to feel she is a nuisance just because there is another form to fill in. Once again she should be offered the full range of modern prostheses to choose from.

RECURRENCE

When a patient's condition changes because of metastatic spread, she may require a change of prosthesis due to her altered size. Here the nurse may need to give advice on a more suitable bra fitting or an alternative style of prosthesis. A new false bosom may be the last thing on the patient's mind, but her morale is of great importance, and at some stage during treatment a lop-sided figure may just be the 'last straw' if left uncorrected.

If a local recurrence should occur and a bra and prosthesis cannot be worn, a comfy may be secured inside a vest or petticoat or over a dressing, and will help to simulate the right shape. This may be a problem the district nurse may be faced with. Once again maintaining morale is a large part of the care of any cancer patient and, even though the patient may be bedridden, she may still like to receive her visitors and will not want to feel embarrassed.

Special problems

Another not so rare problem may be that of the bilateral mastectomy woman. Her first mastectomy may have been performed many years ago when radical surgery was fashionable. Her recent surgery may have been more simple, so that, although she may need the same size of prosthesis, she may not require the same shape on both sides (Fig. 6.4).

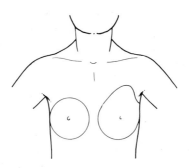

Fig. 6.4   A bilateral mastectomy.

Another problem occasionally encountered is that of the young woman who has been successfully treated for cancer by mastectomy, and is now pregnant. As a pregnant lady's bosom tends to increase in size, she may need additional prostheses to allow for this change both before and after the birth.

Coloured ladies needing a dark prosthesis also present a small problem as at present there are only two companies (Spencer Intermed and Remploy), who provide a brown covering to their prostheses. As yet the demand is not very large and manufacturers do not find it economical to produce brown covers in large quantities, but most of them are willing to help out with individual cases as the need arises.

The need for partial prostheses is growing as many more surgeons are favouring lumpectomy and wide excision as primary treatment for breast cancer. Many of these women will not require any kind of prosthesis, but a few may need to use one to achieve balanced contours. A long-term problem may occur when there has been a weight gain, as the untreated bosom may enlarge, whilst the treated one will remain the same size due to the effects of the radiotherapy. As yet, only one company (Camp) manufactures a partial prosthesis.

Bras, prostheses and swimwear are by no means a problem for every woman, but it is important she should be able to turn to someone for advice. The nurse is in the unique position to be able to offer advice of this nature, as this is as much a part of 'total patient care' as attending to her postoperative needs.

It is important to understand that the patient usually relates more easily to the nurse than to the surgical appliance fitter. It may be the nurse that the patient turns to for advice regarding swimwear and necklines. Many women feel that they are doomed to wearing high-necked clothing, including unattractive swimwear, for the rest of their lives. This should not be so, as today's type of surgery rarely leaves the chest or axilla very deformed, so that a fairly ordinary neckline can be worn with the prosthesis. Some suitable examples are shown in Fig. 6.5 and it is worth remembering that many women continue to wear ordinary swimsuits after their mastectomy.

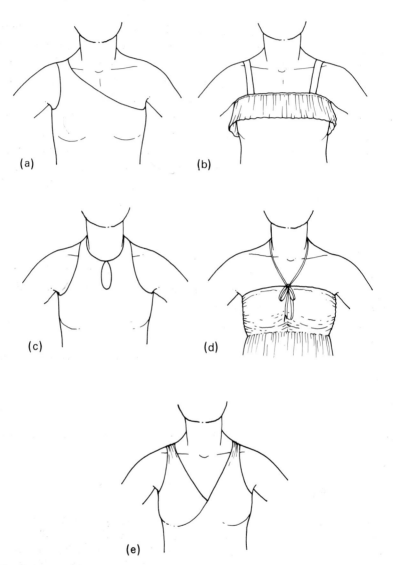

(a)

(b)

(c)

(d)

(e)

Fig. 6.5 Different styles of neckline (a–e) which may be suitable for wear after breast surgery.

Swimsuits with premoulded cups have several advantages; a pocket can be sewn on to the cup to enable the prosthesis to be tucked securely inside. The prosthesis can either be one especially made for the purpose (e.g. Sea-scamp by Camp Ltd.) or the woman may use her own if it is waterproof. (A pocket sewing service is available through the NHS, although the woman will have to pay for this, approx. £4–5 per pocket). Without premoulded cups, it is quite difficult to mimic the shape of the natural breast, especially when flattened by the tightness of the material. The premoulded cup will also prevent an erect nipple showing through. It may be of benefit to the patient if the ward and outpatient department has a catalogue of suitable swimwear selections, and a list of local shops which would be able to help should she encounter any difficulties.

EXERCISE

Katherine wants to return to her family and social life and to her job as soon as possible. Foremost on her mind is 'looking normal', in other words regaining symmetry.

1 What problems might Katherine encounter in relation to both clothing and prostheses?

2 How might the nursing staff help Katherine to solve these problems?

REFERENCE

Downie, P. A. (1974) Cancerous diseases — 1: Rehabilitation. *Nursing Times* **70**, 1276–8.

FURTHER READING

Akehurst, A.C. (1974) Post Mastectomy Morale. *Nursing Mirror* **139**, 66.

Akehurst, A.C. (1975) Symposium on Mastectomy, *Nursing Mirror* **140.**

Andrew & Stanway (1982) Bras. In *The Breast.* Granada Publishing, London.

Lasser, T. (1972) You and the Art of Grooming. In *Reach for Recovery,* T. Lasser & W.K. Clarke (eds). Simon & Schuster, New York.

Pope, B. (1981) After the Mastectomy: Prosthesis and Clothing. *Nursing Times* **77**, 314-18.

Westgate, B. (1980) Breast Prosthesis in the UK (Guide to Types and Suppliers). *Nursing Times* **76**, 1262.

Winkler, A. (1977) Confronting One's Changed Image — Choosing the Prosthesis and Clothing. *American Journal of Nursing* **77** (9) 1433-36.

Chapter 7
Help in Hospital:
Psychological/Practical

Mimi Hondagneu

Breast cancer is the commonest type of female cancer in the Western world. In recent years it has become a frequent topic of discussion in the media, in particular women's magazines. However, in spite of the openness about breast cancer today and information available about treatment methods, this never prepares a woman for the moment when she finds a lump in her own breast. Not only does she fear the possibility of a diagnosis of breast cancer but she may be faced with a potentially mutilating operation.

It is the nurse who spends more time than any other health professional with the patient. For nurses working with breast cancer patients this can be a very rewarding role, for while the patient's physical care needs may be relatively few, her psychological and information needs are great.

Outpatient department

By the time a woman arrives in the outpatient department of a hospital she may have already gone through a series of psychological reactions, including shock, disbelief, or perhaps denial. Her husband or partner may have been through a similar set of reactions, but the fact that they have consulted a doctor means they have begun to confront the thought that something may be wrong. Nevertheless, the news that a lump is or may be cancer can come as a shock.

At this point, the nurse can begin an assessment of the patient and family needs to assist coping mechanisms. It is important to ascertain if the patient has understood what the surgeon has said; her feelings about the diagnosis; if she understands what procedures or tests may be performed; and any specific worries about the illness or operation (Gray 1981). It is useful for patients to know approximately how long they might be in hospital at this point and what limitations will exist in the postoperative period. The woman's husband or partner should be included during these discussions and it should be determined if there are personal problems to be resolved before the woman's hospital stay (e.g. young children at home, an elderly parent, what to tell an employer). Occasionally, a referral to the social worker or a health visitor may be indicated at this point.

Families may be too dazed at this time to absorb much information and it is important to allow their concerns to control the content of the interview. If possible, it is extremely useful that they have the name and telephone number of an informed professional to contact should they have queries prior to admission. For many patients, the period between diagnosis and hospitalisation is more stressful than coming into hospital. Previously unconsidered questions or concerns may plague the mind once the patient returns home and some women find these difficult to share with an already worried family. The opportunity to telephone someone who has professional credibility as well as counselling skills can be a tremendous relief. For these reasons, some hospitals assign these patients a clinical nurse specialist for follow-up.

Preoperative care

Upon admission to hospital, the woman enters an alien world. Due to the age groups most often affected by breast cancer, many women will never have been in hospital except perhaps to bear children some years previously. Whether or not a woman's fears and anxieties are dealt with in the best possible manner is highly dependent on the quality and degree of nursing involvement.

A nursing history and assessment are essential on admission to hospital in planning care and eventual discharge for the individual patient. A patient's adjustment to her diagnosis is determined and affected by many factors: educational, ethnic, religious and social background; past experience of illness and reactions to this; and the available family and social supports (Moetzinger & Dauber 1982). This latter area is an especially important one for nurses to take note of. Several studies have demonstrated that the majority of breast cancer patients receive the most emotional support from spouses, family and close friends (Bullough 1981; Moetzinger & Dauber 1982). Therefore, it seems reasonable to include the patient's most significant person when giving information or advice throughout the hospital stay.

Bearing the above in mind, the nurse should begin by dealing with the patient's chief concerns. Unless the patient can relate her worries and fears and discuss these in an open way, she is unlikely to be able to absorb any information. Each person will bring her own baggage of private fears based on her own past history and current events. For one patient the main concern of the moment may be the anaesthesia, for another the loss of the breast, for another the diagnosis. Each woman is an individual and generalisations cannot be made because of age or marital status.

One vital preoperative assessment is to ascertain the patient's understanding of the procedure to be done. The nurse might say, 'Tell me what you understand is happening tomorrow'. There might be confusion over terminology or incomplete comprehension of the proposed surgery. Due to the anxiety at this time, the patient may not comprehend all that the surgeon has said; therefore, reinforcement of previous information is important.

Physical preoperative care is centred on preparing a clean operative site. The axilla on the affected side should be shaved and the patient instructed to have a bath the evening prior to or morning of surgery. Information needs include how and when the anaesthetic is given; how the patient may feel immediately postoperatively and her right to ask for pain medication; how the dressing will look; the routine use of wound drains and the possibility of waking with an intravenous infusion; and the coughing and deep breathing exercises explained and demonstrated. Both the woman and her husband may be concerned about how the wound will look — it is surprising how many women expect to see a circular, raw wound. Explaining that the chest will appear flat on the operative side and only a horizontal line of stitches visible can allay some anxiety and assist towards the first steps in dealing with a change of body image.

Postoperative care

PHYSICAL

Physical postoperative care problems include prevention of wound infection, observation for haematoma or fluid collection, regaining range of motion in the affected arm, and prevention of lymphoedema (Ahana & Kunishi 1981). Confidence in the nurses' ability to make her comfortable and deal with immediate physical needs inspires trust, and this can help prepare the woman for her first look at the scar (Costello 1970).

PSYCHOLOGICAL

Most studies agree that 80% of women with breast cancer eventually cope with their diagnosis, and that nurses need to assess factors which might interfere with coping ability. These might include problems relating to changed body image, sexual concerns, problems with family or social supports, fear of the diagnosis of cancer and past coping abilities.

BODY IMAGE

Confronting an altered body image will be one of the primary postoperative tasks of the patient. This will of course be dealt with differently by individuals and therefore nursing action is dependent on patient reaction.

It has been stated that attitudes of parents, society, peer groups and significant others are important determinants in how a person will eventually form an image of herself (O'Brien 1980). However, 'awareness of the changing image is not always consistent with the actual physical changes of body image'. Although a woman knows her breast is gone or altered, this may take some time to assimilate. Indications of beginning to cope with an altered body image are:

1   When the patient begins to look at and touch the changed area.
2   When she allows others to look at it.
3   When she begins to ask questions about caring for the area.

4   When the patient begins to take over responsibility for care (Costello 1970, O'Brien 1980).

Thus, it is important for the woman to be encouraged to look at her scar while still in hospital. The woman who delays looking at the wound, is afraid to touch the area, or who seeks no information about self-care, may develop problems in relation to changed body image.

Many women express feelings of mutilation and 'feeling like less of a woman'. In the Western culture, breasts are a symbol of femininity, and the loss of one may indeed be felt as having an effect on one's attractiveness or identity as a woman. Morale in hospital might be considerably affected by encouraging the patient's usual efforts at grooming (Mantell 1982). Wearing make-up, and visiting the hospital hairdresser help emphasise femininity. Fitting the patient with a temporary soft prosthesis under her nightdress returns a missing curve, and encouraging her to dress once drains have been removed de-emphasises the 'invalid' role. After the initial postoperative period, the woman should also be given information regarding the permanent prosthesis. This may be done with printed leaflets, as well as showing her samples of prostheses available. Encouraging such activities should be geared to the individual and timed to her own needs. The patient needs time to discuss feelings that are listened to with empathy (never sympathy) and the preceding suggestions should be viewed as helping the patient back to normality.

All women who have had a mastectomy should be made aware of the Mastectomy Association. This is a volunteer organisation of women who have themselves been through the experience of mastectomy. At their centre in London, a permanent display of brassières, prostheses, and swimsuits may be viewed and up-to-date lists of shops and stockists are available. One may telephone them for information and advice about practical matters, and they are a resource for both lay and professional persons. They also provide printed booklets in conjunction with the Health Education Council, which are useful to give to women both pre- and postoperatively.

The use of volunteers for patients in hospital can be another morale-booster. All the reassurance of family, friends and nurses is useful, but for some patients seeing is believing. The sight of a healthy, well-dressed, well-adjusted woman who has undergone the same surgery says more than all the reassuring words in the world. Sharing practical concerns with someone who has been through them and emerged well-adjusted, can be the patient's best advertisement for hope.

SEXUAL DIFFICULTIES

The most important person to a woman trying to adjust to a changed body image is her sexual partner. Reassurance that she is still attractive and desirable is desperately needed. Maguire (1975) found that a third of the mastectomy patients interviewed experienced sexual difficulties. However, husbands or partners may have their own fears or fantasies regarding either the surgery or the diagnosis. The nurse can discuss these with him and perhaps offer information and guidance in dealing with these problems. A barrier to the couple's functioning may be the husband's concern over his own possible reaction to the wound. One way of dealing with this is to give the husband a description of it and offer to include him during the dressing change. This can effectively help the couple — the patient, because she does not have to decide how to show her husband the wound; and the husband, because the possible initial shock may be overcome in hospital. This should be done only after discussion with both parties, and must take into account the couple's usual pattern of relating. The woman who has never allowed her husband to see her nude would not welcome such a suggestion.

The majority of husbands want to be helpful to their spouses after discharge from hospital, but are uncertain how. Many will refrain from sexual overtures afraid this may physically hurt or offend their wives. The wife may interpret this as rejection — that her husband has lost interest in her or is repulsed by her appearance. The nurse can explain that mastectomy need not interfere with sexual function and emphasise the importance of good communication in avoiding this 'mastectomy bind'. In a couple where communication has always been poor, specialist sexual or marital counselling may be indicated. These problems do not just exist in the event of mastectomy. Some women feel mutilated by the more minor deformity of a wide excision or tylectomy.

FAMILY SUPPORT

Another need in hospital may be the support of family members. Breast cancer affects not only the woman herself but every member of the family to some degree. Previous communication patterns will become apparent in the family interaction. Some families react to the patient's anxiety or distress by trying to minimise or reassure that everything will be fine. They need to understand the importance of allowing the woman to grieve while still giving support. Depression can in fact be a symptom of repressed grief. Not knowing what to say is a common problem. If honest feelings are expressed with difficulty, simple non-verbal gestures can communicate caring. Physical contact such as holding a hand or an arm around the shoulder can demonstrate support.

Family may benefit from knowing that the patient may experience depression or mood swings. Knowing what is normal behaviour and how to react to this is helpful to the woman's rehabilitation. Ignoring a spouse's depression or telling her to 'pull herself together' can result in the patient feeling misunderstood and therefore more isolated (Brand & Van Keep 1978). A husband's encouragement and support can be an important factor in a speedy recovery.

There are many practical things a husband may do to assist in his wife's rehabilitation. Returning to normality as soon as possible is healthy for the entire family. It does not help the woman to be made to feel an invalid. On the other hand, recognition of possible temporary handicaps (e.g. avoiding heavy lifting, fatigue) and assistance with these can convey caring. Encouraging socialising and outings, especially once fitted with the external permanent prosthesis, can help the woman make that first step in coping with the outside world again. If the woman has taken pains with her appearance, it should be recognised — she needs to feel she is still attractive and desirable.

Older children, especially daughters, may need information about how to help their mother. Any daughter over eighteen could be included in a teaching session with her mother about BSE. Women with female relatives who have had breast cancer have a 2–3 times higher risk of developing it than some one without a familial history. Also, women already diagnosed have a 10% incidence of developing breast cancer in the opposite breast (Hubbard 1979). Since most women discover breast lumps themselves, knowing a systematic, purposeful method of self-examination might conceivably lead to earlier detection in a high-risk group.

It is important in teaching BSE to emphasise that the reason for this is to become familiar with how their breasts normally look and feel, so that any change from normal can be reported. It is useful to give the patient and her daughter a printed leaflet as well as demonstration. This exercise might also be a time to air questions the patient and her daughter may have regarding breast lumps and may be a good opportunity of dispelling myths and providing patient as well as family education.

Younger children in the family may require special comfort. Admission of their mother to hospital is certain to alter the family routine and introduce insecurity. Hiding the fact that mother has had a mastectomy can become a secret in the family and children may become anxious through fear of the unknown (Brand & Van Keep 1978). If information can be shared in a simple, matter-of-fact way children can generally accept this. As long as children feel their world is secure and mother has not abandoned them, they need not suffer undue anxiety. When possible, it is helpful if they may visit mother in hospital at a time when she is feeling well, to verify that she is coming home again.

FEAR OF THE DIAGNOSIS OF CANCER

As previously mentioned, each patient has her individual concerns. The majority of patients will share a fear of the diagnosis of cancer. For many people, cancer is synonymous with death, and dying of cancer is believed to be slow, painful, and disfiguring. This can lead to a great deal of sometimes unspoken anxiety and confusion for both parent and family. The psychological reaction to a cancer diagnosis is affected by attitudes and beliefs about malignant disease (Maguire 1975).

In helping them to deal with this fear, the nurse needs to assess the patient and family knowledge and experience of the disease. Have they ever known anyone who had breast cancer? A woman who knows people who are alive and well after mastectomy will undoubtedly have a different impression of the disease than one who, for example, has nursed a relative dying of metastatic breast cancer. Have they ever known someone with any other type of cancer? To many people, all cancers are lumped into one category, and if a woman has known someone who died of, say, lung cancer after diagnosis, she may also fear this to be her fate. Encouraging patients and families to ask questions will reveal areas of information deficit. Answering these simply and honestly is imperative and obvious gaps or errors in desired information should be rectified and discussed with other members of the health team.

The mastectomy site, besides necessitating a change in self-image, is also a reminder that a woman has had and may still have a potentially fatal disease (Maguire 1975). Any unusual physical sensation could be interpreted as a manifestation of the physical presence of disease. The nurse can explain, for example, that numbness along the scar line and on the posterior surface of the upper arm is due to severing of nerves during surgery and that sensation takes a long time to return, and in some cases, never quite returns to normal. 'Pins and needles' or the odd stabbing pain can also occur and, if present, should be explained as being due to the surgical treatment. Lack of energy or fatigue is a complaint voiced by many women after mastectomy, and may continue for a period of months. This varies from individual to individual, but should again be explained as within the norm.

Questions about prognosis or recurrent disease are fraught with anxiety and are always difficult. Health care professionals who work with breast cancer are familiar with trends in the disease; however, no one can predict the future for a particular patient. The answer to a question such as 'will it spread?', must be geared to that individual. The breast cancer patient needs honesty, realistic reassurance, and hope. The nurse should respond with openness, warmth, a sense of caring, and be willing to respond to the experience or need of the present. In addition, practical information should be given, such as explanation of 'routine' procedures and follow-up care. The purpose of various routine diagnostic tests such as bone scans is to detect metastatic disease, and to serve as a baseline for future investigations.

Conclusion

The majority of us go through life without much thought of our own mortality. This issue tends to be confronted in situations such as the death of a loved one or in the diagnosis of a serious illness. Reactions to this vary according to the individual and a variety can be observed in the woman after mastectomy. The result can be positive or negative: negative, in that the threat of death is dwelled on; or positive, in that an opportunity is granted to look at one's life and become aware of what one's priorities are. Counselling of the patient in these times of emotional upheaval is of the utmost importance.

EXERCISE

1 Discuss the term 'body-image'. How might Katherine's body-image be altered? What could be done to help her adjust to her new body-image?
2 What other diseases or operations might alter a person's 'body-image'?

REFERENCES

Ahana, D & Kunishi, M. (1981) *Cancer Care Protocols for Hospital and Home Care Use.* Springer, New York.

Brand, P.C. & Van Keep, P.A. (1978) *Breast Cancer — Psychosocial Aspects of Early Detection and Treatment.* MTP Press, Lancaster.

Bullough, B. (1981) Nurses as Teachers and Support Persons for Breast Cancer Patients. *Cancer Nursing,* June, 221-5.

Costello, A. (1970) Supporting the Patient with Problems Related to Body Image. Reprinted from the Proceeding of the National Conference on Cancer Nursing, USA.

Gray, S. (1981) The Role of the Nurse in the Breast Unit. In *Breast Cancer Management,* R.C. Coombes (ed.). Academic Press, London.

Hubbard, S. (1979) The Nurse's Role is Vital in Early Detection. *Nursing Mirror.* **149,** 18-20.

Maguire, P. (1975) The Psychological and Social Consequences of Breast Cancer. *Nursing Mirror* **140,** 54-7.

Mantell, J. (1982) Sexuality and Cancer. In *Psychosocial Aspects of Cancer,* Cohen (ed.). Raven Press, New York.

Moetzinger, C. & Dauber, L. (1982) The Management of the Patient with Breast Cancer. *Cancer Nursing* **5,** 287-92.

O'Brien, J. (1980) Mirror, Mirror, Why Me? *Nursing Mirror* **150,** 37-8.

Thomas, S. G. (1978) Psychosocial Issues in Breast Cancer. *Cancer Nursing* **1,** 53-60.

Chapter 8
Problems at Home:
Psychological/Practical

Sylvia Denton

In the UK approximately 21 000 women are diagnosed yearly as having breast cancer and 1 in 14 women have the chance of developing this disease at some time in their lives. Together with the diagnosis of this disease comes all the fear a life-threatening disease may produce, plus perhaps the threat of mutilating surgery. The emotions engendered by these aspects often touch every aspect of her life and therefore that of her family and other social contacts. Where appropriate then breast cancer may be seen as a family disease affecting many. It is the most common malignancy in women and the commonest cause of death in the 35–55 year age group.

Rehabilitation of the breast cancer patient should start at diagnosis and therefore, if possible, limit any adverse psychological effects that the diagnosis might have on the patient and her family. Planning care therefore for both admission to and discharge from hospital is essential.

In controlled studies by Maguire *et al.* (1978) and Morris *et al.* (1977) it was found that up to 25% of women suffered moderate to severe anxiety and depression for 1–2 years respectively. Various coping strategies will be adopted by patients according to their immediate priorities and established coping methods. For some it may be denial; for others various stages of anxiety and depression may have to be worked through prior to acquiring a comfortable coping strategy. It is not only established psychological behaviour that may determine reaction to diagnosis, reaction may be greatly affected by present social circumstances and indeed procrastination in seeking help may be a result of these. Greer (1976) demonstrated that coping by means of denial correlated with delay in seeking treatment.

Upon discovery of a lump or any other symptom many women will strongly suspect cancer until it is proven otherwise, therefore it is important for the nurse to appreciate the extreme anxiety experienced by patients prior to positive diagnosis, whilst the various diagnostic procedures are being carried out. Opportunity to discuss and for an explanation of procedures is essential for the patient and, upon confirmation of the diagnosis, this dialogue should continue. Brewin (1977) states that, 'With cancer there are additional difficulties due to deep seated fears of a special kind not encountered in any other disease, even when closely matched in terms of symptoms and prognosis.' He further states that, 'Patients who feel they are not being told enough are often suffering from a feeling of insecurity due, not to insufficient frankness but to lack of sustained professional interest in their symptoms, lack of good care or lack of information.'

Breast cancer often presents itself to the patient by a chance finding of a lump with no preceding debility, thus adding to the feelings of shock and disbelief. There is a Dutch proverb which would appear to aptly describe this: 'Sickness arrives on horseback and departs on foot'. Methods of facilitating this departure in full may not be available at present, but distancing may be achieved and realistic hope should always be maintained.

Patterns of coping often change in patients with the time and events, loss of an important body part has been likened to a bereavement by Colin Murray-Parkes (1972).

COPING STRATEGIES

Preoperative

Between diagnosis and treatment there is frequently a period of extreme anxiety and shock. During this time opportunity should be given to the patient to express these feelings; use should also be made of counselling skills to start to mobilise the patient's own resources to try and cope, using intervention and referral to other specialist disciplines if and when appropriate.

It is of great value for a community nurse or specialist mastectomy nurse/counsellor to visit the woman at home prior to admission into hospital, for frequently she may not have fully understood diagnosis or its consequences; objective assessment and planning for care are also aided by this. It is imperative that the woman should be fully informed so she is able to make responsible decisions since diagnosis and treatment often will rapidly follow the discovery of symptoms by patients as, 'I feel as if I am dreaming and will wake up', or 'I feel I am looking down on all that is happening'. Amidst the shock and anxiety the woman will usually feel far more at ease and in control in her own home, thus enabling her to express any fears and anxieties and thereby working with the aid of a nurse towards rehabilitation. Practical details about treatments may need explanation and any particular problems relayed back to the ward staff prior to admission into hospital. This type of liaison between community and ward staff is of immense help to the patient in that it provides a continuity of care.

Practical help may be necessary to enable the patient to simply enter hospital; there may be young children to be cared for, or infirm old relatives the patient is responsible for.

Changing emotions of the patient may be apparent to the nurse during the home visit. Shock, denial, depression, anxiety and anger are some of the emotions which the patient may both feel and express to the nurse. Patterns of these emotions vary from patient to patient but will hopefully lead to the establishment of a comfortable coping pattern and emotional equilibrium.

Anger expressed by a patient may be particularly worrying for the nurse, but licence to express this emotion and assurance of acceptance of this without any judgement should be given. In this way therapeutic relationships may eventually develop between patient and nurse without feelings of guilt on the part of the patient.

Fears of threat to, and loss of, sexual identity and body image may be expressed by a patient, and those women without partners may be especially vulnerable to these fears, as has been demonstrated by Denton & Baum (1983). Aspirations and hopes for the future are often dashed (temporarily) when facing mastectomy or oophorectomy. Such questions as, 'What chance have I now of finding someone and settling down?' have been heard from women. The nurse should allow the patient to talk through these fears and to refer the patient to other agencies, such as the Mastectomy Association (see Appendix 1) for additional advice, support and help.

Such initial fears of loss of body image may be seen in some women to override those about the disease of cancer and can often inhibit coping mechanisms coming into action and prolong psychological adjustment. Such patients may have increased risk of psychiatric morbidity.

Postoperative

Prior to discharge from hospital, appropriate plans should be made for care, thus enabling optimum chances for full rehabilitation. At this stage again liaison between hospital and community staff is invaluable. It is essential that a patient who has undergone mastectomy should be fitted with a temporary prosthesis and, if possible, be used to wearing this prior to discharge. She will thus have at least some confidence that she looks more or less normal when dressed and leaves the protected environment of the hospital. The woman should have viewed her scar prior to discharge as this can be a very traumatic experience, and note should be taken by ward staff and relayed to those in the community if this has not occurred. It is not unusual for a woman to experience a phase of postoperative euphoria and this may continue and include discharge from hospital. It is again important that if this is observed it is reported to community staff, as often it may suddenly pass, leaving a woman depressed and afraid. Her family may be very dismayed and upset by this sudden change in mood, so support and explanation is often very helpful to them and the patient should this happen.

Financial problems upon discharge due to the nature of this illness may be encountered. Employment may have terminated because of illness, especially if employment prior to diagnosis had been of an insecure nature. Also patients sometimes experience difficulty obtaining employment after a diagnosis of cancer has been made.

This problem may be especially relevant to a single person or one who happens to be the 'bread winner' in a family.

Single women living alone may experience fears for the future — fears of what will happen and how will they cope should their disease progress to the point of their losing independence. Should this occur, it is helpful for the nurse to provide practical information of care available, thus enabling the patient to try and put this fear aside but have a plan as a 'back-up'.

PSYCHOLOGICAL PROBLEMS AND ACCEPTANCE OF PROSTHESIS

As time passes after discharge from hospital, delay in physical recovery may be apparent and, should appropriate clinical investigation prove negative, it may be seen as a demonstration of psychological problems. Sutherland (1967) observed that preoperatively unresolved expectations of injury were present and there was danger of their conversion into the postoperative phase and conviction that injury had taken place.

At 6–8 weeks postoperatively the patient should be fitted with a permanent prosthesis. Care is required in the introduction of prostheses as it is essential that the patient is both psychologically ready to accept these and understands the need for them. Any prolonged and unreasonable difficulty with prosthetics should be viewed by the nurse as possibly indicating that the patient has some psychological problem that is being sublimated and redirected towards the more practical prosthetic aspect. Choice and suitability of prostheses has been dealt with in more depth in Chapter 6.

The nurse must be alert for the patient who tries to be a 'good patient' and desires to conform to what she sees as the expectations of her quick and easy adjustment, thus denying her own feelings.

FAMILY INVOLVEMENT

Where appropriate the early involvement of the woman's family in discussions about the disease and its treatment is of great importance, as noted by Wellisch *et al*. (1978). This involvement may often help in achieving positive gains from a negative situation. Two such examples are a deepening of relationships within a family and re-assessment of real priorities.

It is important to convey to the woman that you are interested in her feelings, thus giving her licence to express these. Patients traditionally expect the nurse to be only interested in the physical aspects of disease and fear they are wasting nurses' and doctors' time in talking of fears and anxieties. In some cases, specialised counselling skills are needed too, but even the most inexperienced nurse must be able to recognise increased fear and stress and report these to appropriate colleagues.

When a patient has had a relative or close friend who has had cancer (and in particular one where disease was not controlled and perhaps even fatal) this can be especially difficult for the patient and produces increased fear and stress and supports the assumption from both patient and her family that this will be the course of her disease. Counselling and help from the nurse can be valuable in helping the woman and her family cope.

FOLLOW-UP AT HOME

Often only once at home does the patient really start to realise and think about what has happened to her; at this point she may seek more in-depth information about the disease and various courses it may take. The sensitive nurse should be able to judge how much information can be tolerated for, although the patient may demand 'the whole truth', this may hide terrible fear. A course should always be taken whereby truth is maintained, yet only that information which can be absorbed by the patient is given; to go beyond this only serves to cause serious stress and may disrupt any normal coping strategies that may be developing.

When following up the patient after discharge, it is important to check how she is sleeping. During this early period after discharge and often for some time later, the woman may experience sleep pattern disturbance and even occasional nightmares. Should this occur with any regularity, further help should be sought after discussion with the woman. This may be one of the manifestations of a depressive illness.

It is important for the community nurse to have knowledge of possible patterns of emotional change a woman may experience, to note any extreme reaction and to monitor this. Increased dependence is one reaction that may occur; initially this is quite natural whilst the woman attempts to regain confidence and learn to cope with the impact of the disease and its treatments.

Discharge from hospital may present a diversity of reactions. For some women it will be a return to a loving family from whence they can draw strength to cope with their broader social circle. For others they may be fearful of rejection, feeling more at ease within what they see as the 'safe environment' of the hospital where they see themselves as being accepted. Some people see cancer as infectious and talk of feeling unclean even after surgery. Women have occasionally been ostracised by others because of these people's fear of 'catching' the disease. Lack of confidence may occur, manifesting itself as an inability to go out of the home, feeling unable to go to a public place, travel or go where there might be crowds. Such fears should be noted and help given swiftly, including specialist help to avoid exacerbation of the problem if appropriate.

Lymphoedema may become a problem and along with this are the psychological stresses it brings to bear. There is great difficulty in hiding the 'tell-tale' signs, the woman may feel her 'secret' is no longer hers to tell only to who she chooses, and this may cause her to avoid socialising. Added to this is the limiting effect it can have on choice of clothing and this can be depressing. Chapter 12 discusses this problem in greater detail.

Where there may have been a previously 'rocky' relationship this new crisis may well cause it to founder. Wellisch *et al.* (1978) reported that, 'Men with a negative view of the relationship before the procedure tended to become more negative after the mastectomy.' They further reported that, 'In terms of psychosocial trauma of mastectomy the man is anything but a detached observer, even if he takes a seemingly distant stance.'

Women who have undergone mastectomy very often feel a lack of confidence when mixing with their own sex; again this is often prompted by feeling degraded as a woman and therefore not as good as their peers.

Inevitably the time will come for the patient to attend hospital for follow-up. This is often a time pre-empted by fear and anxiety and often a time when the woman may experience a regression in the development of any coping strategy she may have developed. Empathy and understanding from hospital staff during these visits is all-important if the fear generated by these is to be alleviated.

Recurrence

The emotional problems associated with adjusting to primary breast cancer may be only compounded with the occurrence of metastatic disease. This is a time when patients may re-refer themselves for help and support if they received this from a nurse either in hospital or in the community whilst undergoing treatment for their primary cancer. This is a time when such an established relationship can be called upon again to offer support and help, if realistic hope and honesty have previously been maintained within the counselling interviews.

For patients where disease has re-occurred within a short time of primary treatment, full recovery from initial psychological problems may not have occurred. Support and constant assessments to detect any psychiatric morbidity which will need referral for specialist help are therefore important during this time of often intense stress for the patient and her family. Patients often express feelings of great disappointment, with such remarks as, 'I was getting on so well and really felt I was on my feet again'. Patients meeting recurrence some time after the initial disease can experience shock and, again, great disappointment, 'I really thought I had kicked the disease'. Metastatic disease for some women is worse than the initial diagnosis. Close contact between nurse and patient is most important during this time to allow the patient to express her feelings and the nurse to evaluate both the nursing care and especially the patient's emotional needs.

SIDE-EFFECTS OF TREATMENT

Radiotherapy, chemotherapy and the endocrine therapies are those therapies usually employed in the treatment of metastatic disease, and these often have quite unpleasant side-effects. The nurse should always be available to lend explanation and support through these additional traumas for the patient. Chemotherapy may produce nausea, vomiting, alopecia and malaise, and courses of the drugs involved often have to extend over many months. Therefore, practical help as well as emotional support is important. Patients may need to continue employment during this time, thus planning around the drug schedule is important if the patient experiences side-effects, so as to facilitate the minimum absence from work. It is not uncommon for women to experience depression during the course of chemotherapy and they understandably come to dread attending for administration of their drugs as time goes on.

Endocrine therapies often add to the woman's feelings of threat to her sexual identity, some of these causing sudden and abrupt end to menstruation. Radiotherapy may cause psychiatric morbidity; it can have the effect of causing fatigue and general debility, especially towards the end of the treatment regime and for a few weeks after.

Thus recurrent disease and all the implications this has for the patient, together with the treatment often necessary to try and alleviate disease, may cause anxiety, stress, and additional psychological morbidity.

OTHER CONSIDERATIONS

Whilst caring for women who have breast cancer, the nurse should not fail to consider the quality of life these women enjoy. It is important for the nurse to know where the limitations of her expertise are within the psychological context of care and when referral should be made to another specialist discipline for treatment. These specialist resources are essential and the nurse should know how and when to use them and referral should be easily implemented.

It is important to realise that every patient is unique, that each brings to the situation an individual set of priorities, values and past experiences, and that each will then need individual counselling according to these. Sutherland (1967) affirms the value of, 'a warm supportive person whom the patient could trust'. A nurse involved in the care of a patient over a prolonged period may well provide this role, both for the patient and her family. Wellisch *et al.* (1978) states that the psychosocial effects of breast cancer and mastectomy extend in a ripple effect from the patient to her spouse and ultimately to the entire family. This fact must always be taken into consideration when planning and evaluating care. Counselling is one skill the nurse may use in this case of the breast cancer patient, from diagnosis of disease and during treatment for all stages of disease. The British Association for Counselling states that, 'The task of counselling is to give the client an opportunity to explore, discover and clarify ways of living more resourcefully, and toward greater well-being.'

Patients' needs should always dictate the nature of the care delivered. Mara Flaherty (1980), herself a cancer patient, stated, 'I see nurses and patients as strong allies against cancer'. This alliance of necessity may have to be active during prolonged treatment and hopefully prove to be of value in the fight against the psychological aspects of breast cancer.

EXERCISE

Katherine had no opportunity to discuss her disease and possible operation between the time she discovered the lump in her breast and the time she was admitted for surgery.

1   Discuss the feelings Katherine might have had prior to hospital admission and how a nurse might have alleviated some of them.

REFERENCES

Brewin, T. B. (1977) The Cancer Patient: Communication and Morale. *British Medical Journal* **2**, 1632.

Denton, S. & Baum, M. (1983) Psychological Aspects of Breast Cancer. In *Breast Cancer,* Margolese, R. (ed.) Churchill Livingstone, Edinburgh.

Flaherty, M. (1980) Living with Cancer, In *Cancer Nursing Update:* Proceeding from the second international Cancer Nursing Conference, R. Tiffany, (ed.), Baillière Tindall, London.

Greer, H. S. (1976) Psychological Correlates of Breast Cancer. In *Risk Factors in Breast Cancer,* B. Stoll (ed.). Heinemann, London.

Maguire, P. *et al.* (1978) Psychiatric Problems in the First Year after Mastectomy. *British Medical Journal* **1,** 963.

Morris, T., Greer, H. & White, P. (1977) Psychological or Social Adjustment to Mastectomy. *Cancer* **40,** 2381.

Murray-Parkes, C. (1972) *Bereavement Studies of Grief in Adult Life.* Pelican Books, London.

Sutherland, A. M. (1967) Psychological Observations in Cancer Patients. *Institute of Psychiatric Clinics* **4,** 72.

Wellisch, D. K., Jamison, K. & Pasnau, R.O. (1978) Psychosocial Aspects of Mastectomy II: The Man's Perspective. *American Journal of Psychiatry* **135,** 543.

Chapter 9
Nursing Care: Radiotherapy

Recent advances in radiotherapy have placed a great responsibility upon the nurse, both in the outpatient department and the community. She is required to care for her patient, to support their relatives, and also to have specific expert knowledge in the treatment of cancer and the management of radiotherapy. She will have to dispel myths which have grown over half a century. Reports of hair loss and vomiting are quite common, though in many cases inappropriate with today's modern technology.

Currently, radiation therapy has three specific applications in breast cancer treatment.

1 As primary treatment, where the radiotherapist offers radiation as the first choice of treatment whether it aims to be curative or palliative, or when the patient refuses surgery.

2 As an adjunct to mastectomy or local excision to ensure that all the cancer cells are killed — this is sometimes known as an 'insurance policy', or to alter the hormonal status, i.e. radio-oophorectomy.

3 As palliation to relieve pain caused by distant metastases.

Let us look at the category of primary treatment. The patient may present with a large lump without evidence of metastatic spread. Her condition could be treated with radical radiotherapy in the first instance, though other modalities of treatment such as hormone or chemotherapy may also be employed. The aim is to shrink the cancer and kill off the cells before they have a chance to fungate or metastasize. This can be achieved either by teletherapy alone or, in certain circumstances, by insertion of iridium wires to the tumour (Fig. 9.1). The aim therefore is said to be curative. Should a similar circumstance present itself where metastatic spread is evident, then breast radiation would be performed in order to hold the tumour in check and to prevent fungation. The metastatic disease would also have to be monitored (if causing no symptoms) and treated at some stage of the disease.

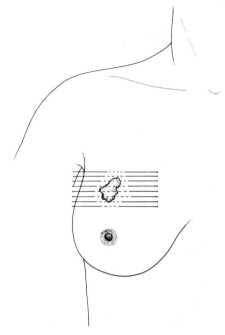

Fig. 9.1   Radioactive wires which deliver a high dose of radiation directly to the tumour.

A woman who presents with a fungating tumour may or may not have evidence of spread, as one of the curious facts about breast cancer is that locally advanced disease does not always indicate that the tumour has disseminated. The aim here is to dry up the mass and hopefully shrink the cancer so that it does not fungate again. Radiotherapy has proved to be quite successful in these cases, as the odour and exudate are cleared up quite quickly, and in many cases regression of the tumour is evident (*see* Chapter 13).

So what of the care of these patients? Once again we have to remember that we are dealing with a woman and her family who have just been told of the diagnosis of cancer; unlike the women who have undergone mastectomy, the woman has not had three or four weeks to get used to the idea before reaching the radiotherapy department. As irradiation is at the beginning of her programme of treatment, she will probably want to know as much about her disease as she does of her impending treatment. A woman who has undergone surgery has had a week or so in a hospital bed with nurses in constant attendance, of whom she could ask questions about her cancer and management. Here in a busy clinic, she has a limited time with her consultant, and probably a few minutes with a nurse. The patient then has to face a bewildering world of a busy clinic, whilst trying to 'take in' instructions regarding tests and treatment sessions. It is little wonder that the patient becomes frightened and confused.

How can the nurse minimise such a bewildering experience for her patient? Firstly let us look at what, in general, this patient's requirements are:

1   To gain information about her disease.

2   To know about any tests which may be required throughout the treatment.

3   To understand the aim of her treatment, how long it will last, and what will happen after that.

4   To know about the side-effects of treatment.

The first requirement may be handled in several ways, but one of the most effective methods is to involve the husband (or significant other) in the interview with the consultant, as a partner will generally remember the points the patient forgets. This, however, can be a time-consuming process, and the nurse may have to explain in more detail what the consultant has said.

In the same way the second point can also be handled by involving the partner. In many instances it is the nurse who will provide details of the tests ordered by the doctor. Often in the bluster of a busy department, information for such procedures is lacking in detail, as the nurse often has to divide her time between this frightened patient and the next. Her few brief words therefore have to be very carefully chosen. This point can be illustrated by the following:

'The consultant wants you to have an ultrasound examination, I've booked it for you, it's at 10.00 a.m. on Friday 27th. You will have to go to the second floor.' Or 'We have booked an ultrasound for you, the test doesn't hurt, there are no needles involved and it shouldn't take longer than half an hour.'

Whilst both of these explanations are informative, the first one simply iterates what is on the appointment card. The second example is a little better, though how much more information can be retained by the patient at this stage is debatable. A simple written explanation of such tests, either printed on the back of the appointment card or on a separate sheet of paper would be of much more use. The woman can then take it home and absorb the information at her leisure. This is not meant to replace any verbal information being given to the patient, but merely to supplement and reinforce what has been said.

It is the responsibility of the consultant to ensure that the patient understands the aim of the treatment. However it is often the nurse who has to explain in more detail about the actual therapy. It helps enormously and saves much worry and confusion if the nurse accompanies the patient to the appointments desk, makes the appointment with her, and takes her along to the waiting area she is expected to report to. A brief word can be mentioned about the machine and how long the patient will be in the treatment room each day. The nurse can also mention that regular blood tests will be performed on certain days, when the patient will be detained for longer than normal. The patient also needs to know how long the treatment is planned for. All this seems time consuming but it is quite justified, as it is both worthwhile in terms of patient cooperation and courteous to show the patient around the department in which she will be spending the next six weeks or so. The future management should be discussed with the consultant with the nurse present, so that she can clarify any points with her patient at a later stage if necessary.

The last point is probably the most time consuming, though undoubtably the most important. A balance has to be struck between telling the patient of every conceivable side-effect, and gliding over the main ones in order to minimise them. Ideally a quiet room should be found to have this discussion before treatment commences. It is a time for a patient's worries and fears to be discussed, so that the nurse can reassure her and allay her fears. Side-effects common to all forms of radiotherapy (such as lethargy and low blood count) can be covered and myths surrounding radiation therapy dispelled.

Myths and misconceptions

Points on which the nurse can reassure the patient include: 1. Nausea is not usually associated with radiotherapy to the breast. 2. Radiotherapy will kill the sweat glands very quickly so the axilla will not produce an odour. 3. The hair loss in the axilla may re-grow at a later stage.

PRIMARY TREATMENT

For the patient undergoing primary treatment by radiotherapy, there may be the additional fear that the cancer is still inside them — they feel somehow unclean since no surgery has been performed to remove the lump. This is particularly the case with the lady who presents with a fungating tumour, as her problems are obvious — a smelly open ulcer which exudes constantly. Hope of 'cure' is usually unreasonable; at best, the lesion will dry up, skin will grow over the ulcer and the problem will be temporarily halted, but there can be no guarantee of abolishing the disease itself. If these patients are admitted for their treatment, they should be encouraged to engage in ward activities with other patients, as they often feel reluctant to do so. The obvious problem of odour may be dealt with by using a charcoal backed dressing. The patient's room can be made odour free by the use of commercial air fresheners, as the woman is often acutely aware of the smell of the lesion and may discourage visitors from calling.

There is no reason why she should not dress, nor is there any reason for her to look lop-sided if the ulceration has engulfed the whole breast and left the chest wall flat (*see* p.38). Should a small area of ulceration occur in a large-breasted woman, she would be well advised to buy a couple of sleep bras in order to provide some support during the day, if she is unable to wear her ordinary bra. There are no specific instructions regarding arm care for these patients as each case is individual and must be guided by both the radiotherapist and physiotherapist.

If the patient is being treated as an outpatient it is wise to mobilise the help of the community services, such as the district nurse and the social worker, who can ascertain whether other agencies such as Meals-on-Wheels or Home Help are necessary.

ADJUVANT TREATMENT

The second category of patients who are having radiotherapy as an adjunct to surgery have different needs. As radiotherapy usually starts four weeks after surgery, the patient has had a few weeks in which to start to accept her disease, and women will present at the clinic displaying varying degrees of this acceptance. The nurse will have recognised some of these emotions in her patients which may range from acceptance to denial, conflict and hopelessness. Being aware of the pattern of gradual acceptance and coping can help the nurse to direct more time to the women who are displaying less ability at coping than their counterparts.

These women have usually had some time to find out about radiotherapy treatment before attending the clinic, thus making the job a little easier for the outpatient nurse. However the task then falls to the ward nurse, which may prove difficult for many reasons. As results from paraffin sections are not known for approximately eight days after the operation, the doctor may not be able to inform the patient that radiotherapy is indicated until the day before she is discharged, which leaves the nurse with very little time to explain the treatment. Even more of a problem are the patients who have their surgery on a 'five-day ward'. They have the added problem of having to recover physically and emotionally in four days before going home, so that information on practical points and further treatment will not be absorbed. These patients need extremely careful follow-up in the outpatients or suture clinic in cases where radiotherapy is indicated, therefore thorough liaison between the ward, outpatients and radiotherapy clinic is essential if patients are not to 'fall through the net'. A similar problem occurs if the radiotherapy department is located in another hospital. If the ward is not able to give information because it is inappropriate or unavailable, or simply due to lack of time, the outpatient nurse should be aware of this and be ready to continue the information-giving process for her patient. In many enlightened hospitals, the nurses from the ward also work in outpatients on a rota basis, thus ensuring some level of continuity of care.

For the patient who has had a wide excision, radiotherapy will usually be given to whole breast and axillary area to a maximum of 60 grays (6000 rads). Physical care is discussed on p.93, however the psychological needs may vary. She may feel lucky to still have her bosom, or desperately unlucky to have had breast cancer in the first place. Once again the nurse can identify the woman who is in need of more help.

Women who have had a mastectomy may not have radiotherapy to the scar or chest area, but may require treatment to the axilla, superclavicular nodes and/or internal mammary chain in order to attack the adjacent lymph nodes (Fig. 9.2). These patients usually need quite a lot of emotional support as it can seem to them that they have the 'worst of both worlds'.

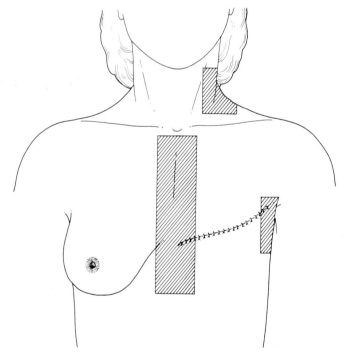

Fig. 9.2   Possible areas of irradiation.

SUMMARY

Here is a summary of some of the common needs and problems of patients undergoing radiotherapy to the breast, either as primary or adjuvant therapy.

Problem.   Skin care — general.
Action.   No perfumes, deodorants, soap or talcum powder (except Johnson's baby powder) to be used.
Wash with warm water and pat dry with a soft towel.

Problem.   Skin care — neck.
Action.   Avoid stiff or starched collars.
Wear soft silk/polyester scarves as protection from sun and wind.
Use fabric softeners when washing clothes.

Problem.   Skin care — axilla.
Action.   Avoid restricting clothing.
Avoid synthetic and harsh materials.
Expose to the air as often as possible.
If moist desquamation occurs, this can be treated by applying, e.g. hydrocostisone 1% or Gentian Violet as prescribed by the doctor.

Problem.   Skin care — breast/scar and ribcage.
Action.   Bra should be removed if causing pressure — remember to tell patient that she can secure temporary prosthesis into petticoat/vest. Special cotton-backed prostheses are available (Spencer Banbury).

Problem.   Ink marks showing.
Action.   Advice on clothing, e.g. wear soft silk scarf or roll-necked jumper.
Warn patient that ink marks may be applied when radiotherapy is planned.

Problem.   Lethargy.
Action.   Explain that this is quite normal.

Advise extra rest in afternoons if possible. Ensure adequate sleep at night if this is a problem, refer to doctor who may prescribe a sedative.

Enquire if patient is unduly worried about anything in particular, and refer to appropriate person if necessary.

Make sure she goes for her blood tests.

Refer for Home Help if required.

Problem.   Lack of appetite.

Action.   Explain general points about good nutrition — suggest small meals three or four times a day.

If too tired to cook suggest convenience foods and ready cooked meats.

Check no dysphagia (if internal mammary chain or superclavicular nodes treated).

Ensure good oral hygiene, Mucaine suspension often prescribed.

Problem.   Respiratory problems: acute — some inflammation of mucosa and dry cough.

Action.   Can be treated with codeine linctus if prescribed.

Problem.   Respiratory problems: latent — pneumonitis breathlessness.

Action.   Reassure that this can and will be treated — antibiotics and steriods usually prescribed. Relief can be obtained by inhalations of tincture of benzoine.

Problem.   Respiratory problems can lead to permanent pulmonary fibrosis.

Action.   If this is diagnosed patient will need help in coming to terms with this new development. Advice given as to limitation of activities.

Problem.   Arm movements — may become limited.

Action.   Encourage patient to use arm normally.

Early referral to physiotherapist essential.

Problem.   Arm movements — stiff shoulder.
Action.   Inform doctor so he can refer for immediate treatment by physiotherapist if indicated.
Nurse should be aware of exercises prescribed.

Problem.   Oedema.
Action.   Usually temporary in nature at this stage. Encourage normal use of arm movements. Restrict heavy lifting.
Elevate arm on pillows whenever possible.

This chapter has aimed to look at the use of radiotherapy as in the treatment of breast cancer and some of the more pertinent aspects of nursing care. The subject of radiation therapy for patients suffering from disseminated disease has not been dealt with, as it was felt that this could be more adequately covered in the chapter on metastatic disease.

EXERCISE

Following her modified radical mastectomy, the surgeon referred Katherine to a radiotherapist. The radiotherapist recommends that Katherine undergo a six week course of radiotherapy to her left axilla in order to ensure that all malignant cells in that area are destroyed.
1   How can the nursing staff minimise Katherine's anxiety about her radiotherapy treatment?
2   What problems or possible problems might Katherine encounter as a result of the radiotherapy treatment? How can the nursing staff prepare Katherine for these?

FURTHER READING

Baker (1979) Implants and Applicators. Scan 10. *Nursing Times* **75,** 37–40.
Cole M. P. (1964) The Place of Radiotherapy in the Management of Early Breast Cancer: A Report of two clinical trials. *British Journal of Surgery* **51,** 216.
Dostal E. R. & Elder L. E. (1979) Breast Cancer: Special Nursing Considerations. *Journal of Practical Nursing* **29**(4), 16-18, 45.
Fisher B. (1970, 1972) Postoperative Radiotherapy in the Treatment of Breast Cancer — Results of the NSARP Clinical Trial. *Annals of Surgery* 711-30.
Greer S. (1979) Psychological Consequences of Cancer *The Practitioner* **222,** 173–8.

Ramirez G. (1975) Combined Chemotherapy/Radiotherapy as an adjuvant to Mastectomy in Patients with positive nodes (Abstract). Proceedings of the American Association for Cancer Research **62**, 224.

Sandland R. (1978) The Nature of Radiotherapy. In *Oncology for Nurses and Health Care Professionals,* vol. 1 'Pathology, Diagnosis', R. Tiffany (ed.). Allen & Unwin, London.

Sandland R. (1978) The Role of Radiotherapy. In *Oncology for Nurses and Health Care Professionals*, vol. 1 'Pathology, Diagnosis', R. Tiffany (ed.). Allen & Unwin, London.

Smith T. (1981) *Further Treatment. Breast Cancer.* Gerald Duckworth, London.

Toombs M. E. (1978) Nursing Care Study, Breast Cancer. (Domiciliary Care Following Radiotherapy). *Nursing Times* **77**, 279-80.

Tully J. P. & Wagner B. (1978) Breast Cancer: Helping the Mastectomy Patient Live Life Fully. *Nursing* **8**(1), 20-5.

Webb P. (1979) Nursing Care of Patients Undergoing Treatment by Teletherapy. *Cancer Nursing Vol. 2. Radiotherapy,* R. Tiffany (ed.). Faber and Faber, London.

Chapter 10
Nursing Care: Chemotherapy

The rationale behind the use of chemotherapy is based on the principles of normal cell growth (*see* Chapter 2). A knowledge of cell growth and behaviour helps the nurse to understand why and how chemotherapy works and why side-effects occur. Each cytotoxic drug acts in certain ways and in knowing how each drug works we also can predict any adverse effects which are likely to occur; as nurses we can then take steps to prevent or alleviate these effects. Let us examine:
1   How cytotoxic drugs work.
2   Cell kinetics and how this determines how and when to give cytoxic drugs.
3   The cytotoxic drugs most commonly used to treat breast cancer.
4   Side-effects of these cytotoxic drugs and the nursing actions which might prevent or alleviate these.

CYTOTOXIC DRUGS

How cytotoxic drugs work

In cancer tissue as well as in normal tissue, individual cells will be in differing phases of the cell cycle at any one time. Some will be in the G_1 phase, some in the synthesis phase and so forth. Some potentially dividing cells will be temporarily out of the cell cycle, lying dormant in the G_0 phase waiting for the right stimulation to send them back into the cell cycle. Studies carried out on the effect of radiotherapy on cell activity showed that sensitivity of cells to irradiation was different in different phases of the cell cycle (Tubiana 1971).

Chemotherapists have also tried to determine whether there was a difference in sensitivity of the cell to cytotoxic drugs in different phases of the cell cycle. What was found was that cytotoxic drugs fell into one of two groups. One group of drugs included those which

97

appeared to be highly toxic to cells depending upon which phase of the cell cycle they were in. These were termed *phase-specific drugs*. The second group of drugs were those in which the phase of the cell cycle made no difference to the toxicity of the drug. In other words, the drug was as toxic to the cell in one phase as it was in any other phase. These drugs are called *cycle-specific drugs* (Table 10.1). This was a radical change from the traditional way of classifying cytotoxic drugs (Table 10.2).

Table 10.1   Some cycle-specific and phase-specific cytoxic drugs (kinetic classification of cytotoxic drugs).

Cycle-specific	Phase-specific
Nitrogen mustard	Cytosine arabinoside
Phenylalanine mustard	Vincristine
Chlorambucil	Vinblastine
Cyclophosphamide	Methotrexate
Busulphan	Bleomycin
Thiotepa	Procarbazine
5-Fluorouracil	Asparaginase
Actinomycin-D	
Mitomycin-C	
Mithramycin	
Adriamycin	

It was also found that not all phases of the cell cycle last for the same length of time. Some phases, especially the G_1 phase, vary a great deal. Some cells have no G_1 phase while other cells have G_1 phases which last up to 30 hours or more. It appears that slow-dividing cells (normal and tumour) have long G_1 phases while fast-dividing cells (normal or tumour) have very short or no G_1 phases. It was also once believed that all cancer cells grew and divided very quickly, while all normal cells grew more slowly than cancer cells and this belief previously provided the basis for the way in which

Table 10.2   Traditional classification of cytotoxic drugs.

Alkylating Agents
e.g. nitrogen mustard, phenylalanine mustard, cyclophosphamide

Antimetabolites
e.g. methotrexate, 5-fluorouracil

Vinca alkaloids
e.g. vincristine, vinblastine

Antimitotic antibiotics
e.g. adriamycin, bleomycin, mithramycin, mitomycin-C

Miscellaneous drugs
e.g. procarbazine, asparaginase

chemotherapy used to be given. Thus the whole question of how tumours grow needed to be re-examined. Part of the difference has to do with the fact that normal cells divide to replace cells which have died while cancer cells divide and multiply to add to existing tumour population. Cancer, then, is not a mass of rapidly dividing cells as was previously thought. Rather, it is a mass of cells which are dividing at the normal rate but because the mass fails to lose cells in the normal fashion, the tumour cell population is constantly increasing and so is the size of the tumour.

Both phase-specific cytotoxic drugs and cycle-specific cytotoxic drugs will only kill cells which are in the cell cycle. They do not act on cells which are in the dormant G_0 phase (or temporarily out of the cell cycle).

How and when to give drug therapy

Chemotherapy is most likely to be successful when the number of tumour cells is at its smallest. For this reason, chemotherapy for solid tumours is most effective when given immediately after the bulk of the tumour has been removed, usually by surgery. This approach is not as widely used for patients with breast cancer for several reasons.
1   Traditionally, breast cancer has been viewed as a local disease. Surgery and radiotherapy were seen as the best way of treating it.
2   Side-effects of many of the cytotoxic drugs effective for breast

cancer were such that it was thought to be unnecessarily cruel to subject patients who had already undergone mutilating surgery to side-effects such as hair loss.

3   Studies have shown that many breast tumours are hormone-dependent and therefore some form of hormone manipulation has been used instead of chemotherapy (*see* Chapter 11).

4   Lack of resources and personnel both in wards and outpatients departments have made it impossible in many centres to administer cytotoxic drugs on such a large scale.

5   Lack of data about the long term effects of cytotoxic drugs.

How and when to administer

Historically, one of the early ways of administering cytotoxic drugs was by the use of one drug on a continuous basis. This was termed a *single agent regime* and arose from the old belief that tumour cells divide and reproduce more rapidly than normal cells. It was thought that by using a single agent continuously, the patient's blood level of the drug would remain constant and, although some of the patient's normal cells would be affected, the cancer cells would be more affected because they were growing more rapidly. This type of chemotherapy regime is now seldom if ever used. New understanding of cell kinetics (mentioned previously) has enabled new regimes to be established which could be as effective or even more effective with less toxicity to the patient.

Combination chemotherapy

For many malignant conditions, including breast cancer, a combination of cytotoxic agents was found to be successful in treating the disease, using the minimum number of drugs to achieve the maximum therapeutic effect. Two drug combination chemotherapy was tried which attempted to use two drugs which killed tumour cells but which had different side-effects. This would increase the action against the tumour without increasing toxicity to any one particular site, such as bone marrow.

Intermittent chemotherapy

Skipper (1964) found firstly that doses of cytotoxic drugs do not kill a set *number* of cells but rather a fixed *percentage of cells*. Secondly, if you increase the dosage, you increase the percentage of cells killed. Thirdly, that normal cells could quickly repair the damage done to them by cytotoxic drugs while cancer cells, which grow at a fixed rate even after cytotoxic drug administration, did not repair the damage done to them as quickly. These and other studies led to a new concept of cancer chemotherapy which is called intermittent high dose chemotherapy based on the kinetic cell theory. High doses of combination chemotherapy are given with periods of rest in between. During this time, normal tissue recovers fairly quickly from the side-effects of the drugs, while cancer cells recover fairly slowly. Using this type of chemotherapeutic regime, the tumour cell population gradually gets smaller and smaller until, hopefully, it disappears. A comparison between the different methods of giving cytotoxic agents can be seen in Figs. 10.1 and 10.2 using the same doubling time graph as was found in Chapter 2.

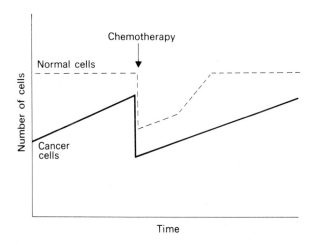

Fig. 10.1   Single course chemotherapy and its effect on cells.

It can be seen from Fig. 10.1 (single course chemotherapy) that normal cells are growing and regenerating at the same rate as they are dying so the total number of cells remains constant. The tumour cell population, however, is constantly increasing because, although tumour cells are increasing, none are dying. When a single course of treatment is given, both the total number of normal cells and the total number of tumour cells decreases. But the tumour cells are not totally eradicated. So normal cells regenerate fairly quickly to make up the number lost through treatment and over a period of time tumour cells also recover and continue to grow. If no further treatment is given, the tumour cell population will eventually increase to such a size so as to kill the patient.

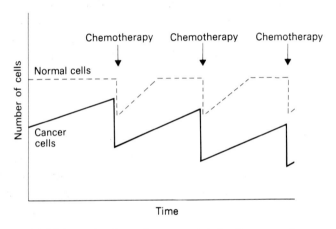

Fig. 10.2   Multiple course chemotherapy and their effects on cells.

In Fig. 10.2 we see that the first treatment affects normal and tumour cells in the same way as in Fig. 10.1. After a short rest period, normal cells regain their correct level while tumour cells increase slightly but not to their pretreatment level. Thus, when the next treatment is given after the prescribed rest interval, the percentage of tumour cells decreases even further. Treatment continues until all signs of disease are gone.

With intermittent high dose chemotherapy, care must be taken to carefully monitor the recovery of normal cells and to allow the correct time to pass before the next treatment. If the treatment intervals are too short, normal cells do not have a chance to recover and the next treatment can cause too great a drop in normal cell population; this could prove as fatal to the patient as the disease itself. Equally, too long an interval between treatments can allow the tumour cell population to regenerate to its pretreatment level; the therapeutic effect of the treatment is thereby lost.

Drugs commonly used

It is not the intention of this chapter to include in any detail the specific drug protocols for breast cancer. In specialist centres new drugs and drug protocols are constantly being subjected to clinical trials, and changes in drugs can occur quite quickly. For this reason, this section will deal with the main cytotoxic drugs used in breast cancer and will describe how they act, explain both the traditional and the kinetic classification in which they are placed, and discuss the specific side-effects of each drug.

ADRIAMYCIN

In the traditional classification of cytotoxic drugs adriamycin is an antimitotic antibiotic. In the kinetic classification, it is a cycle-specific drug. Adriamycin is useful in treating many of the solid tumours and is especially successful in treating breast cancer. It forms part of nearly all the established protocols for the treatment of breast cancer. The specific side-effects of adriamycin include gut toxicity, bone marrow suppression, stomatitis (e.g. mouth ulcers), severe alopecia and cardiotoxicity. Adriamycin is also excreted in urine and can often change the colour of urine to red.

CYCLOPHOSPHAMIDE

In the traditional classification of cytotoxic drugs, cyclophosphamide is an alkylating agent. This means that its chemical structure contains an alkyl (chemical formula CH_2) which combines with other compounds to change the structure of DNA. Although the drug was designed to act selectively against cancer cells to minimise side-effects, studies have shown that this is probably not what happens. Cyclophosphamide was thought to act in the presence of certain enzymes which are found in high quantities in tumour cells. It is a widely used cytotoxic drug and forms part of many breast cancer chemotherapeutic protocols. In the kinetic classification of cytotoxic drugs, cyclophosphamide is a cycle-specific drug which means it acts on cancer cells equally in any part of the cell cycle.

The most important side-effects of cyclophosphamide are bone marrow suppression, alopecia (this tends to be dose related), gut toxicity and irritation to the lining of the bladder where it is excreted, causing a chemical cystitis.

METHOTREXATE

Methotrexate is a drug which is traditionally classified as an antimetabolite. Metabolites are those compounds which come together and make up the DNA in the cell nucleus in the presence of certain enzymes. Antimetabolites inhibit these enzymes, thus making it impossible for DNA to replicate. In the kinetic classification of drugs, methotrexate is a phase-specific drug and is most toxic to the S phase of the cell cycle. Methotrexate acts as a folic acid antagonist. Folic acid is a vitamin essential for normal cell growth. The enzymes in the nucleus of the cell change folic acid into folinic acid where it is used by the cell for growth. Methotrexate has a structure similar to that of folic acid and binds with the relevant enzymes, thus rendering the enzyme inactive. This prevents folic acid from changing into folinic acid and thus cell growth is halted. Unfortunately, it is not only cancer cells which have their folinic acid supply destroyed by methotrexate. All folinic acid in every cell, normal or tumour, is destroyed. This gives rise to many side-effects such as gut toxicity, severe mouth ulceration and bone marrow toxicity. To prevent or minimise these side-effects, there is a way to stop the activity of methotrexate in the body after it has effectively destroyed the reproducing cancer cells. To do this, folinic acid is given 12–24 hours after the methotrexate has been given, which replaces the folinic acid destroyed by the dose of methotrexate. In short, the methotrexate is in the body long enough to act against tumour cells and then its action is reversed by giving folinic acid in order to minimise or prevent the side-effects.

VINCRISTINE

Vincristine is classified traditionally as a vinca alkaloid. These are organic compounds whose effectiveness as cytotoxic agents was discovered accidently when vinca extracts from the periwinkle plant were being tested as hypoglycaemic agents. They turned out to have no effect on blood sugar levels but it was noticed that they caused a marked drop in the white cell count. Vincristine was one of the extracts used in this study. The precise action is not fully known or understood but it was initially found to stop cell division at a particular stage of mitosis. More recent studies have shown that vincristine may even work earlier in the cell cycle than the mitosis stage and in fact may halt cell DNA replication in the S phase. In the kinetic classification, vincristine is called a phase-specific drug. Although some leucopenia (decreased white cell count) is known to be a side-effect of vincristine, the drug is relatively free of bone marrow toxicity. This makes it a very useful drug to use in combination chemotherapy with drugs that are toxic to bone marrow. In this way two drugs can be used to fight the breast cancer cells without the side-effect of being doubly toxic to the bone marrow.

5-FLUOROURACIL

5-Fluorouracil — or 5-FU as it is commonly called — is classified traditionally as an antimetabolite (*see* p.104 for an explanation of the action of antimetabolites). Uracil is one of the metabolites found in RNA, the protein which assists in DNA replication. Without RNA, there can be no DNA replication. Uracil appears to exist in greater quantities in tumour tissue than in normal tissue. 5-FU has a chemical structure similar to uracil and so it is taken up by the tumour tissue as if it were uracil. Then the cytotoxic properties of the drug act on the tumour which has taken it up, causing tumour cell death probably by destroying the enzyme responsible for joining the uracil to the chain of RNA. Side-effects include nausea and vomiting, bone marrow depression, mouth ulcers, gut toxicity, some hair loss, skin reaction especially in strong sunlight and also discoloration of veins after prolonged use of the drug. This manifests itself as brown lines on the skin following the path of the veins up the arms.

Miscellaneous drugs

There have been other drugs used with some success on certain patients with breast cancer. Phenylalanine mustard (Melphalan), an alkylating agent in the traditional classification of drugs and a cycle-specific agent in the kinetic classification of drugs, is one such drug. Although primarily used in the treatment of other solid and systemic malignancies, some specialist centres are using Melphalan in the treatment of some patients with advanced carcinoma of breast. High-dose Melphalan is sometimes used as a last line of treatment in conjunction with bone marrow transplant. In these cases patients are screened to determine if there is metastatic disease in their bone marrow. If the marrow is clear of disease, plans are made to remove large quantities of bone marrow from the patient whilst under general anaesthetic. Melphalan is then injected intravenously in a high dose which kills the malignant cells present in the body. In doing so, however, the remaining bone marrow becomes completely suppressed. Shortly after this, the bone marrow previously removed from the patient is returned to the patient and by the process of cell recognition returns to the marrow site. Here it begins to reproduce and regrow to replace the marrow destroyed by the Melphalan. This procedure presents many actual and possible nursing problems which are discussed on p.112.

NURSING CARE

In order to assist nurses to plan nursing care for patients receiving chemotherapy, this section is designed in two parts. The first part identifies many of the common side-effects of drugs which can cause problems for women undergoing a course of chemotherapy. The relevant nursing action for each actual or potential patient nursing problem is presented. The second part of this section identifies which problems from the first part are applicable to each of the drugs and identifies other problems specific to each drug.

Common patient nursing problems

With many cytotoxic drugs used in treating patients with breast cancer patient nursing problems may arise. The goals or aims of care are:

— to prevent side-effects
— to alleviate those which are unavoidable
— to enable the patient to cope with side-effects during the course of treatment
— to enable the patient to carry out normal daily activities once treatment is finished.

Problem.   Hair loss.
Action.   Prepare patient, husband, partner and/or family. Be sure to emphasise that hair will re-grow after treatment is completed.
Order wig if patient wishes to have one.
Provide suggestions and advice about suitable hair coverings as an alternative to a wig such as scarves, turbans or hats.
Help patient to concentrate on hobbies or activities to distract her from dwelling on herself.
If facilities are available in unit/hospital, offer her the 'scalp cooling' technique to prevent hair loss (*see* p.113).

Problem.   Nausea and vomiting with accompanying anorexia due to gastric disturbance.
Action.   Give antiemetics as prescribed especially before meals.
Evaluate with patient the effectiveness at each meal time.
Ensure that she is sitting comfortably at meal times.
Keep the bed and locker area tidy and well ventilated.
Give and encourage mouth washes and oral hygiene after meals.
Offer light, appetising meals, using small portions when the patient feels able to eat. Assess food preferences and encourage family to bring in what food the hospital cannot provide.
Measure and record amount of vomit as well as fluid intake to prevent/minimise possible dehydration.

Problem.   Risk of infection due to low white blood cell count due to bone marrow depression.
Action.   Teach patient appropriate mouth care and encourage mouth care especially after meals.
Teach patient to avoid cuts, burns and scratches. Report any that do not heal to medical staff.
Monitor and report any rise in temperature.

Teach patient to avoid others with infections. If an inpatient, place in a bed away from any one who may have an infection.

Problem.   Tiredness and lethargy due to low haemoglobin from bone marrow depression.
Action.   Explain the possibility of this occurring to patient.
Encourage planned rest periods in the day to fit in with patient's daily living activities.

Problem.   Possible bleeding due to thrombocytopenia from bone marrow depression.
Action.   Observe for signs of bleeding from gums, urine, etc. and report any abnormal bleeding.
Explain this possibility to patient. Teach her to report any abnormal or spontaneous bruising.
Avoid giving injections except when necessary. Apply pressure to injection site for 3–5 minutes.

Problem.   Sore mouth due to damage to mucosal lining from drug.
Action.   Examine mouth carefully each day for dryness, bleeding or ulcers.
Encourage good oral hygiene with an antiseptic mouthwash especially after meals. Use a soft toothbrush to avoid damage to gums.

Specific patient nursing problems

PATIENTS RECEIVING ADRIAMYCIN

In view of the effects and side-effects of adriamycin the following care plan might be appropriate for the woman who is receiving this drug, in addition to all the problems discussed previously.

Problem.   Urine may turn bright red causing *anxiety*.
Action.   Explain this possibility to her and that it will go away in 24–28 hours.

Problem.   Possible chest pain or palpitations due to cardiotoxic effect of the drug.
Action.   Explain that she will have a heart test (ECG) prior to treatment and why.
Explain what an ECG is.
Teach patient the importance of reporting any chest pain.

Other special considerations

Adriamycin can cause severe necrosis and tissue breakdown if the drug for some reason comes out of the vein and into the tissue which surrounds that vein (extravasation). If this should occur the nurse should *immediately* apply ice to the site. Medical staff must then prescribe hydrocortisone cream to be applied for 24 hours. Extravasation of adriamycin is a very uncomfortable and painful experience for the patient and this side-effect must be treated with great immediacy as patients have been known to suffer permanent damage following extravasation to an area, often necessitating skin grafting.

Patients receiving adriamycin sometimes experience a feeling of hotness or pyrexia. If this happens, the temperature should be recorded at regular intervals — such as four-hourly — and antipyretic nursing measures taken, such as use of fans and removing heavy bedclothes. Patients can also experience a feeling of warmth and see a red line following the path of the vein whilst having adriamycin administered. Although little can be done to prevent this from happening, anxiety can be largely allayed by explaining beforehand that this sometimes happens and will disappear after the drug treatment has finished.

PATIENTS RECEIVING CYCLOPHOSPHAMIDE

The nursing action in response to the risk of infection, weakness and lethargy, and nausea and vomiting to patients receiving cyclophosphamide are as discussed in the previous section. Two other problems occur in addition.

Problem.   Hair loss. (Hair loss associated with cyclophosphamide is dose related and only occurs in about 50% of patients.)
Action.   Scalp cooling technique (p.113) has *not* yet been proved effective for this drug.

Problem.   Chemical cystitis because cyclophosphamide is excreted in the urine and can irritate bladder lining.
Action.   Explain the possibility of this occurring to patient and the need for adequate hydration to prevent this.
Devise a fluid intake regime with the patient to ensure a daily intake of 2–3 litres daily. Provide fluids which the patient prefers or encourage relatives to bring them in.

PATIENTS RECEIVING METHOTREXATE

For patients receiving methotrexate the problems and actions are similar to the other cytotoxic drugs discussed.

Problem.   Nausea and vomiting.
Action.   *See* p.107.

Problem.   Sore mouth (*see* p.108).
Action.   Give folinic acid as prescribed. Explain about taking folinic acid at home and its importance to the patient.

Problem.   Possible rectal bleeding due to gut irritation from methotrexate.
Action.   Explain the possibility of this happening to the patient. Observe stools for blood and teach patient to observe and report any blood.

Long-term side-effects

Methotrexate is known to have a long-term bone marrow toxicity which can produce delayed lethargy and tiredness, infection, or bruising and bleeding (*see* p.108). This possibility should be discussed with the patient in order that she might not be unduly anxious should any of these occur and should be able to recognise and report any of these side-effects.

PATIENTS RECEIVING VINCRISTINE

With the effects and side-effects of vincristine, the following care plan might be appropriate.

Problem. Tingling and numbness in hands and feet (peripheral neuropathy).
Action. Explain the possibility of this occurring to the patient. Teach her to observe and report this.
Ensure that reflexes, especially ankle jerk, are tested before each treatment.

Problem. Constipation due to neuropathy in nerves supplying the gut.
Action. Explain the possibility of this occurring, to the patient. Ask her to observe and report evidence of constipation.

Problem. Sore mouth, nausea and vomiting.
Action. *See* pp.107–8.

Problem. Hair loss (*see* p.107).
Action. At the moment there is no evidence to indicate that scalp cooling will be effective against hair loss in patients having vincristine.

Other effects

As with adriamycin, vincristine can cause tissue breakdown and necrosis if extravasation occurs. Precautions should be taken to prevent this, but should it occur, the same measures as described previously should be taken.

PATIENTS RECEIVING 5-FLUOROURACIL

This agent, 5-fluorouracil, shares the following common problems of chemotherapy: risk of infection, tiredness and lethargy, possible bleeding, sore mouth, and nausea and vomiting. *See* pp.107–8 for suitable nursing actions.

Problem.   Diarrhoea due to gut toxicity.
Action.   Explain the possibility of this occurring to the patient and encourage her to report any occurrence.
Give kaolin compounds to prevent/treat diarrhoea.

Other effects

This drug has a minor effect which could be distressing to the patient unless she is aware that it might occur: it can cause darkening of veins which presents as a brown line on the skin following the path of the vein. For this reason no one vein should be used continually if at all possible when giving this drug. This problem occurs more frequently in patients who are dark-skinned.

PATIENTS RECEIVING MELPHALAN

Melphalan shares the following problems with other chemo-therapeutic agents: hair loss, nausea and vomiting, high risk of infection, extreme tiredness and lethargy, high risk of bleeding, and sore mouth.

Because melphalan, especially given in high doses, causes far more severe side-effects than many other drugs, the above problems are much worse than in patients receiving other cytotoxic agents. These patients are nursed in pathogen-free environments with the strictest reverse barrier nursing precautions. It takes about two weeks for the bone marrow to begin to reach a near normal level and, during that time, the patient is practically depleted of red and white blood cells and platelets. High doses of intravenous antibiotics are given to prevent/treat infection and intravenous fluids are given continually to prevent dehydration. This is a very dangerous and distressing time for the patients and relatives and a high priority of nursing care must be to keep the patient and her relatives completely informed of progress; give simple but honest explanations beforehand and be available to relatives to listen to their anxieties. The two weeks immediately after the melphalan injection and replacement of bone marrow will be frightening ones when the patient will be very ill indeed. It is during this time that careful monitoring and care are essential.

Scalp cooling

Loss of hair through chemotherapy is one of the most distressing effects of cytotoxic drugs. Over the past two decades various efforts have been made to try to prevent hair loss (alopecia) from occurring. Early attempts involved the use of forehead tourniquets to decrease the blood supply to the scalp. These, however, proved to be ineffective.

In 1979 a trial was carried out at the University of Arizona in the United States into the use of scalp cooling as a means of preventing hair loss from the drug adriamycin. Results were quite favourable and many ways of effectively cooling the scalp were tried. A more recent study at the Royal Marsden Hospital (Anderson 1981) has reported significant decrease in hair loss with scalp cooling in patients receiving adriamycin. Most of the patients in this scalp cooling trial were, in fact, patients with carcinoma of the breast. It was also found that patients with no liver metastases had little or no hair loss after receiving adriamycin and that the amount of hair loss was dose-related in that the higher the dose, the greater the risk of hair loss. Other centres have begun to use scalp cooling routinely for patients receiving adriamycin and other cytotoxic agents known to cause alopecia. Although there are small variations in the actual technique, the principles of scalp cooling as a means of preventing alopecia remain the same.

At least a quarter of an hour before the chemotherapy is given the patient thoroughly wets her hair. A wet crêpe bandage is sometimes wound round the patient's head after this. Over the wet bandage, or on the wet hair itself, is placed an ice cap of some description. These caps are now being made commercially by one or two firms but were originally hand made for the purpose of the trial at The Royal Marsden Hospital from hot/cold packs taped together and molded into the shape of a head before being placed in a freezer. The cap is secured firmly onto the head by means of a dry crêpe bandage. Centres differ as to the length of time the scalp should be cooled prior to giving the chemotherapy but the range seems to be between 10 and 30 minutes. After the chemotherapy has been given, the cap is kept in place for at least half an hour, although different centres vary as to this length of time. After the prescribed time, the cap is removed and the patient is given a towel and hair dryer to dry her hair.

There are one or two mildly unpleasant side-effects of scalp cooling, notably headache and dizziness. These are prevented or alleviated through careful care of the patient during the procedure. The patient should be lying comfortably in a quiet place or sitting in an arm chair, preferably one that reclines. She should also be encouraged to remain on the bed or in the chair for a short time after the procedure to minimise or prevent dizziness and headache.

EXERCISE

Katherine might be classed as a breast cancer 'success story' as she has been disease free and living a normal life for a good number of years now. Let us look at another patient with different problems requiring different medical and nursing management.

Evelyn is a 52-year-old publican's wife who had a left simple mastectomy nearly ten years ago. She has had follow-up appointments in the outpatient department of her local hospital since her mastectomy and has remained completely well. Recently, however, she has noticed some lumps in her axilla and went to her GP. He referred to the local hospital and the surgeon asked the medical oncologist in the hospital to see Evelyn. The oncologist recommends a course of chemotherapy and arrangements are made for Evelyn to come to the hospital every three weeks for chemotherapy which involves the use of the following drugs: adriamycin and cyclophosphamide.

1 Write a plan of care for Evelyn which takes into account the physical, social and psychological problems which she might encounter as a result of treatment.

REFERENCES

Anderson, J. (1981) Scalp Hypothermia in the Prevention of Doxorubicin-induced Alopecia. In *Cancer Nursing Update,* R. Tiffany (ed.). Baillière Tindall, London.

Skipper, H.E. *et al.* (1964) Experimental Evaluation of Potential Anti-cancer Agents. *Cancer Chemotherapy Reports* **35**, 3–11.

Tubiana, M. (1971) The Kinetics of Tumour Cell Proliferation and Radiotherapy. *British Journal of Radiology* **44**, 325–47.

FURTHER READING

Dean, J., Salmon, S. & Griffiths, K. (1979) Prevention of Doxorubicin-induced Alopecia with Scalp Hypothermia. *New England Journal of Medicine* **301**, 1427–8.

Hill, B. T. & Price, L. A. (1978) Some Principles of Cancer Chemotherapy. In *Oncology for Nurses and Health Care Professionals,* R. Tiffany (ed.). Allen & Unwin, London.

Price, L. A. & Hill, B. T. (1978) The Role of Chemotherapy. In *Oncology for Nurses and Health Care Professionals,* R. Tiffany (ed.). Allen & Unwin, London.

Priestman, T. J. (1980) *Cancer Chemotherapy: An Introduction.* Montedison Pharmaceuticals, Barnet.

Chapter 11
Nursing Care: Hormone Therapy

Hormones play a large part in the growth of normal breast tissue as well as in malignant change. The effect of hormones on breast cancer has only been fully appreciated in recent years and many types of manipulation of the hormone environment are being assessed in women with breast cancer. In the light of this, let us consider:

1   Outline of hormones which affect the breast and breast cancer.
2   Primary endocrine therapy in breast cancer.
3   Secondary endocrine therapy in breast cancer.

Hormone therapy (or hormone manipulation) is another systemic way of treating breast cancer. Patients are seldom, if ever, cured by this form of treatment but the aim is to slow the disease process, not merely to prolong life but to improve the quality of life.

Not all patients will respond to hormone manipulation. Powles (1978) estimates that 30% of patients with metastatic breast cancer will respond to hormone manipulation through some kind of endocrine therapy. Patients with slow growing tumours (the rate being measured by the interval between the time of primary diagnosis and the time of diagnosis of metastases) usually respond to hormone therapy, while those with rapidly growing tumours (such as those who have metastases at the time they present with a primary tumour) usually do not respond quite so well. The location of the metastases will also affect the response to hormone manipulation: those with bone metastases respond better than those with liver metastases. Younger women (aged 20–35) and women over 60 appear to respond better to hormone therapy than those women who are middle aged.

Oestrogen receptors

Studies have shown that some tumours contain oestrogen receptors. Circulating oestrogen is picked up by these receptors and causes the tumour to grow. Tumours can be tested for absence or presence of oestrogen receptors through a special laboratory staining technique. In normal breast tissue oestrogen stimulates the growth of the lactiferous ducts. Tumours which arise in these ducts are more likely to be stimulated to grow by circulating oestrogen.

Priestman (1980) provides a long list of information regarding oestrogen receptors in breast tumours, some of which are summarised here.

1 Between 60 and 70% of primary breast tumours contain oestrogen receptors. These tumours are said to be *oestrogen receptor positive*. In metastatic breast cancer the percentage of oestrogen receptor positive tumours is slightly lower.

2 Premenopausal women tend to have a *lower* percentage of oestrogen receptor positive tumours than do postmenopausal women.

3 A tumour which is oestrogen receptor (abbreviated ER) positive can produce metastases which are ER negative, that is, metastases which do not contain oestrogen receptors, and vice versa.

4 Some tumours may have sections which are ER positive and sections which are ER negative.

5 The more oestrogen receptors found in a tumour the more likely that tumour will respond to hormone therapy.

6 Between 50 and 70% of ER positive tumours will respond to hormone therapy while only between 5 and 10% of ER negative tumours will be sensitive to hormone therapy.

To understand the types of hormone therapy used to treat breast cancer it is important to understand which hormones act on the normal breast. Hormone therapy involves either altering the hormone environment or totally removing certain hormones from the body. Fig. 11.1 shows the hormones which act on the breast.

HORMONES FROM THE ANTERIOR GLAND

The pituitary gland is situated below the hypothalamus at the base of the brain and is responsible for the majority of hormone activity in the body. It is divided into two: the anterior part and the posterior part. The hormones secreted by the anterior part have the greater

effect on the breast; they are:
    Adrenocorticotrophic Hormone (ACTH),
    Thyroid Stimulating Hormone (TSH),
    Growth Hormone (GH),
    Follicle Stimulating Hormone (FSH),
    Luteinising Hormone (LH).

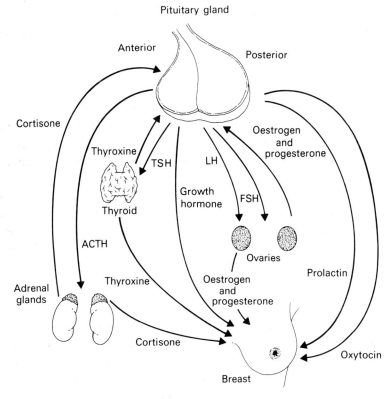

Fig. 11.1   Hormones which effect the breast.

ACTH

ACTH is the hormone which stimulates the adrenal glands to produce the steroid hormones, the most important of which is hydrocortisone. Hydrocortisone affects all basic tissue metabolism including breast tissue metabolism, and is essential to life. The adrenal glands also produce small amounts of oestrogen and progesterone. When hydrocortisone is released from the adrenal glands into the circulation, the level of hydrocortisone determines how much more ACTH needs to be released from the anterior pituitary. When hydrocortisone levels in the blood drop, the low level stimulates more ACTH to be produced. When the level of hydrocortisone in circulation is satisfactory, little or no ACTH is produced. This phenomenon of body chemistry is known as the *feedback mechanism* and continuously regulates nearly all hormone levels in the body.

TSH

TSH stimulates the thyroid gland to produce thyroid hormones such as thyroxine and tri-iodothyronine. These hormones are responsible for regulating metabolic rate in all tissues, including breast tissue. The level of thyroxine is regulated by a negative feedback mechanism where the thyroxine levels in turn tell the pituitary gland to either secrete more TSH or stop secreting TSH. When levels of thyroxine are high, the pituitary stops producing TSH; when they are low the pituitary secretes more TSH. Thyroxine also affects the way growth hormone acts on breast tissue. This will be discussed in the next paragraph.

GH

GH is produced by the anterior pituitary and is responsible for tissue growth. It acts directly on the individual tissue, such as breast tissue, and is not regulated by a feedback mechanism. Instead there seem to be outside factors which affect the amount of growth hormone: genetic factors, diet, absence or presence of other metabolic disorders, absence or presence of other chronic disorders, congenital or acquired skeletal disorders, lack of thyroxine. Adequate levels of thyroxine are essential for growth hormone to work properly.

FSH and LH

FSH and LH are also secreted by the anterior pituitary and both act on the ovaries, although at different times and in different ways.

These hormones also work on a negative feedback mechanism. FSH stimulates the ovary to produce a Graafian follicle at the beginning of the menstrual cycle. This follicle produces oestrogen which enters the bloodstream and circulates throughout the body. Following ovulation, the Graafian follicle undergoes changes and becomes the corpus luteum. This corpus luteum produces progesterone whose function is to prepare the lining of the uterus for the possibility of a fertilised egg, or for menstruation should fertilisation not take place. Oestrogen is also responsible for the formation of lactiferous tissue in the breast.

HORMONES FROM THE POSTERIOR PITUITARY GLAND

Prolactin and oxytocin

Produced by the posterior pituitary, prolactin and oxytocin are concerned with the formation and secretion of breast milk following childbirth. Prolactin stimulates the production of milk in the breast and is not regulated by a feedback mechanism. The mechanical action of the infant suckling stimulates the production of oxytocin which causes the milk to be released from the breast.

PRIMARY ENDOCRINE TREATMENT

The term *primary* in this instance does *not* indicate that hormone therapy is being used as a means of first line treatment in breast cancer. For the most part, hormone therapy is restricted to use in women as adjuvant treatment following surgery where some form of spread (usually to the lymph nodes) has been detected or as treatment for women who have developed metastatic involvement several years after surgery was carried out. However, studies are also being carried out in several centres using prophylactic hormone therapy adjuvant to surgery in random samples of women who have not shown evidence of metastatic spread. Primary hormone therapy is carried out differently for different women depending on menopausal status.

Premenopausal women

The most important factor in the decision to treat breast cancer with hormone therapy is the level of circulating oestrogen in relation to the menopausal status of the women. Prior to menopause the ovaries are active and are producing large quantities of oestrogen. For this reason, removal of the ovaries is carried out to remove circulating oestrogen. Bilateral oophorectomy is the surgical removal of the ovaries and is advantageous in that the oestrogen levels drop instantaneously. The operation also affords the surgeon the opportunity to examine the inside of the abdomen and pelvis to see if there is any evidence of metastatic spread.

Patients who are unfit for such surgery or for whom surgery is otherwise contraindicated can undergo a course of radiotherapy to the ovaries. This destroys all ovarian tissue and induces what is known as 'radiation menopause', effectively stopping the production of oestrogen. The advantage of this is that the woman is not subjected to yet another mutilating operation. The disadvantage is that the oestrogen levels decrease gradually over the course of treatment which could be dangerous if the tumour is a fast-growing, oestrogen-dependent tumour. The nursing management of the long- and short-term effects of ovarian ablation will be discussed later in this chapter.

Postmenopausal women

Postmenopausal women generally have low levels of circulating oestrogens because their ovaries are slowly ceasing to produce it. Some oestrogen is present in that a small amount of it is produced by the adrenal gland. If metastatic disease has occurred in postmenopausal women it is thought that the decrease in oestrogen brought about by the menopause might be causing the tumour to grow. In these women, it is sometimes felt that, by giving additional oestrogens, one can shrink metastatic growth. Women with bone secondaries are seldom given oestrogens because it is known to cause hypercalcaemia in these women. This complication will be discussed in Chapter 13.

SECONDARY ENDOCRINE THERAPY

The term *secondary* in this instance refers to women who have experienced a relapse of their disease after previously responding to some form of hormone therapy. Women who have responded to primary hormone therapy, such as bilateral oophorectomy, are more likely to respond to secondary hormone therapy.

Adrenalectomy

The cortex of the adrenal glands is responsible for producing and secreting corticosteroids. As mentioned previously, some oestrogen (and also some progesterone) is also produced by the adrenal glands, and it has been found that premenopausal women who previously have responded to oophorectomy as primary endocrine therapy respond well to adrenalectomy as secondary endocrine therapy. The same is true for some postmenopausal women. Adrenalectomy seems to be especially useful in patients with painful bone secondaries and many women experience rapid pain relief following adrenalectomy even if there has been no clinical decrease in the spread of their disease. For this reason alone adrenalectomy must be seen as an effective palliative form of hormone therapy.

The disadvantage of adrenalectomy is that, in surgically removing these glands, the production of corticosteroids — which are essential for life — is stopped. For this reason, women who have undergone surgical adrenalectomy must receive steroid replacements (i.e. cortisone acetate, hydrocortisone, prednisolone) for the rest of their lives. Even if it is later discovered that adrenalectomy has not succeeded in stopping metastatic spread, the woman still needs steroid replacement therapy for ever. Adrenalectomy is a serious operation. It can be carried out via abdominal approach or loin approach and it subjects the woman to yet another operation.

In the past few years attempts have been made to use drugs to inhibit the production of corticosteroids by the adrenal glands. A first attempt was to administer large doses of cortisone in an attempt to inhibit the production of ACTH by manipulating the negative feedback mechanism. It was thought that large doses of cortisone would stop the pituitary from producing ACTH, which would then stop stimulating the adrenal gland. This treatment proved unsuccessful.

More recently, however, a new drug called aminoglutethimide has been developed and tried in some hospitals. This drug blocks the synthesis of corticosteroids in the adrenal gland. Studies at The Royal Marsden Hospital have shown that, in some patients, aminoglutethimide initiates a similar response in patients as does surgical adrenalectomy without surgery being necessary. An added advantage is that the effect is reversible — while patients take aminoglutethimide tablets they must also take steroid replacement tablets; but, if and when the aminoglutethimide is stopped, normal adrenal function returns and the patient does not have to receive steroid replacement therapy for the rest of her life. A further advantage is that it involves no hospitalisation and there are none of the surgical risks. For these reasons, aminoglutethimide often provides a more appropriate alternative to surgical adrenalectomy in many patients.

Recently, trials have been started in some centres to determine whether aminoglutethimide is useful to prevent metastatic spread and some patients are being given prophylactic aminoglutethimide immediately after mastectomy.

Hypophysectomy

Hypophysectomy, or removal of the pituitary gland, was once a common form of secondary endocrine therapy. It is rarely used now but it is worthy of mention in this chapter because many patients still present with metastatic spread of breast cancer who previously underwent hypophysectomy. It was never a successul treatment for patients with bone secondaries. Patients who have undergone this operation, or who have had pituitary ablation with radiotherapy, will not produce some of the essential stimulating hormone needed for other endocrine glands to work, such as ACTH and TSH. For this reason patients who have undergone this operation will require both cortisone and thyroxine replacement therapy for life.

Androgens

Some postmenopausal women with bone secondaries respond to male hormones usually in the form of a drug called Durabolin. Androgen therapy does not carry with it a risk of hypercalcaemia as does oestrogen therapy and is of particular benefit in treating women with bone marrow secondaries. It is often used, in this instance in conjunction with chemotherapy.

Progesterones

Various compositions of progesterone (i.e. norethisterone and medroxyprogesterone) have been used to treat metastatic breast cancer as a secondary form of endocrine therapy. Unfortunately, it does not have a particularly good success rate. A small response has been found in using progesterone therapy in the treatment of recurrences in the chest wall and in nodules of soft tissue.

Antioestrogens

Antioestrogens are synthetic preparations which are chemically similar to oestrogens but have little oestrogen activity. The most popular antioestrogen in use is called tamoxifen. The function of antioestrogens is to attach themselves to oestrogen receptors (p.117) in tumour cells, thus preventing real oestrogen in the body from binding to these oestrogen receptors and encouraging tumour growth. Antioestrogens do not cause tumour growth when they bind to oestrogen receptors in the tumour. In postmenopausal women, antioestrogens act as cytotoxic agents to the tumour cells. This makes antioestrogen therapy a particularly useful form of secondary endocrine therapy for older women who may not be able to tolerate ordinary chemotherapy.

Recently, trials have been carried out in several centres using tamoxifen as a prophylactic measure and administering these tablets immediately after mastectomy in the early stages of breast cancer to see if it prevents the development of metastatic spread. The effects of tamoxifen as a way of preventing metastases in the early stages of breast cancer have yet to be analysed.

Corticosteroids

Corticosteroids are used mainly for symptom relief in women with metastatic spread of disease. Using corticosteroids has been found to reduce bone pain, pruritis from skin lesions and cerebral irritation due to raised intercranial pressure from brain secondaries. The relief, however, tends to be short lived. These, and other types of metastatic symptom, are discussed in greater detail in Chapter 13.

PERIMENOPAUSAL PATIENTS

Women who are in the middle of the menopause respond poorly to endocrine therapy and it is difficult to predict which form of hormone therapy is best. This is due to the uncertainty of their own hormonal state. Often oophorectomy and adrenalectomy are carried out simultaneously to remove all oestrogens but the results tend to be poor.

SUMMARY OF ENDOCRINE TREATMENT

Endocrine therapy is a particulary successful means of symptom control for some women with metastatic breast cancer. Only recently have trials been carried out using aminoglutethimide and tamoxifen as prophylactic forms of endocrine therapy. In many women, endocrine therapy improves quality of life by decreasing many of the symptoms of the disease spread.

The prime indication for endocrine therapy appears to be age, in relation to menopause, and location of the metastatic spread. Younger women and older women with bone secondaries and whose tumours are slow growing appear to do well on endocrine therapy, while perimenopausal women and those women with faster growing tumours tend to respond better to chemotherapy.

NURSING MANAGEMENT

For those women undergoing either surgical oophorectomy or radiation oophorectomy as primary endocrine therapy, the following patient problems and related care should be considered.

Problem.   Induced menopause leading to sterility.
Action.   Nurses must make sure that both patient and husband/partner understand the implications of this. If *radiation oophorectomy* — contraceptive measures must continue for at least six weeks until sterility actually occurs.

Problem.   Induced menopause leading to dry vagina causing painful and difficult sexual relations.
Action.   This must be carefully explained and advice about lubrication creams given where appropriate.

Problem.   Induced menopause leading to discomfort due to hot flushes.
Action.   Explain to patient that this will happen, offer advice about avoiding tight fitting clothing and the need to sit and rest when hot flushes do occur.

Problem.   Induced menopause leading to mood changes and feelings of loss of femininity.
Action.   Explain to the woman that the menopause often causes mood swings.
Be available to listen to her if she wants to talk about her feelings and worries.
Include husband/partner in discussions if appropriate. Encourage her to emphasise her other feminine attributes (face, hair, clothes).

Patients who are receiving oestrogen therapy may experience different problems and side-effects of treatment:

Problem.   Nausea and vomiting due to change in hormone balance.
Action.   Explain the possibility of this occuring to her. Offer antiemetics and monitor their effectiveness.

Problem.   Shortness of breath due to possible fluid retention from added oestrogens.
Action.   Monitor respiration rate daily or more frequently if breathing problems develop.
Monitor fluid intake and output or weigh daily.

Problem.   Vaginal bleeding due to hormonal changes.
Action.   Advise the patient of the possibility of this happening beforehand and explain that it is only temporary.
Supply sanitary towels as needed. Record estimated amount of blood loss.

If hypercalcaemia develops as a result of oestrogen therapy as can sometimes happen, additional problems will arise and additional nursing care will be required. This will be discussed in detail in Chapter 13.
Patients who undergo either surgical adrenalectomy or medical adrenalectomy (with aminoglutethimide) will experience different problems and symptoms:

Problems.   Unable to cope with physical stress (from an operation or infection) due to absence of natural corticosteroids.
Action.   Explain the need for steriod replacement and the importance of not forgetting to take them, reporting any illness or infection so that dose may be increased, if necessary.
Give patient 'steroid card' and instruct them to carry it at all times.

If taking aminoglutethemide:

Problem.   Possible skin rashes.
Action.   Explain that this is a possible side-effect and that it will only last a week or so.
Give antihistamines if prescribed to stop itch and irritation. Offer calamine lotion as well if desired.

Problem.   Possible occasional headache.
Action.   Explain that this might happen and that it is also only temporary. Offer mild analgesia if prescribed.

Problem.   Tiredness and lethargy.
Action.   Explain that this is a possible side-effect of the drug and that it also is only temporary.
Encourage her to plan rest periods for herself at home to minimise tiredness.

Patients undergoing treatment with androgens will experience an entirely different range of problems and side-effects and need other nursing actions to help them through these problems or symptoms:

Problem.   Androgens cause masculine traits: facial hair, body hair around nipple and increased pubic and axilliary hair, deepening of voice.
Action.   Your patient needs sensitive explanation of the possibilities of these.
Practical advice about hair removal from face and body.
Help her to focus on feminine aspects such as hair style and clothing.

Problem.   Extreme anxiety and loss of femininity due to all of the above.
Action.   She needs someone to listen to her and allow her to talk about these fears and anxieties.

EXERCISE

Evelyn has finished the menopause a few years ago and consequently the treatment which is suggested to her is bilateral adrenalectomy. With reference to the problems or possible problems which might arise following this operation, write a plan of care for Evelyn for her postoperative period.

REFERENCES

Powles, T. J. (1978) Endocrine Therapy. In *Oncology for Nurses and Health Care Professionals,* R. Tiffany (ed.). Allen & Unwin, London.
Priestman, T. J. (1980) *Cancer Chemotherapy: An Introduction.* Montedison Pharmaceuticals, Barnet.

FURTHER READING

Diggory, G. (1978) Care of Patients Receiving Hormonal Therapy. In *Cancer Nursing: Medical,* R. Tiffany (ed.). Faber and Faber, London.

Health Education Council (1975) *The Change of Life.* HEC, London.

Hoover, R., Gray, L. *et al.* (1976) Menopausal Oestrogens and Breast Cancer. *New England Journal of Medicine* **295**.

Hutton, J. (1978) Oestrogens After the Menopause. *Midwife, Health Visitor and Community Nurse* **14**(5), 140-2.

Kushner, R. (1975) *Breast Cancer.* Harcourt, Brace and Jovanovich, New York.

MacMahon, B. & Feinleib, M. (1960) Breast Cancer in Relation to Nursing and Menopausal History. *Journal of the National Cancer Institute* **24**, 733-53.

Phillips, A. & Rakusen, J. (1978) *Our Bodies Ourselves.* Penguin, London.

Smithers, D. W. (1952) Cancer of the Breast and Menopause. *Journal Fac. Radiologist* **4**, 89-96.

U.S. Dept. of Health, Education and Welfare (1979) *The Breast Cancer Digest.* USDHEW, Bethesda, Maryland.

Chapter 12
Lymphoedema

Lymphoedema can be an extremely distressing condition. At best, it is an embarrassment to the woman, as having one arm larger than the other provokes comment. At worst, it can be disabling, interfering with everyday living to such a degree that aids are required in order to function. Pain associated with lymphoedema, either from the anterior thoracic nerve being compressed or from frozen shoulder is extremely difficult to deal with, and can be a source of misery and frustration for both the woman and her family.

The exact cause of lymphoedema is not really known, nor is it fully understood why some women fall victim whilst others escape. The reasons for the delay of onset in some women are similarly obscure at present.

We can look at some of the predisposing factors to help us to predict who is more likely to suffer from lymphoedema as a result of having breast cancer and treatment. Firstly, women who do not have any surgical interference of the axilliary lymph glands (i.e. those who have had a simple mastectomy) are most unlikely to fall victim to this condition, so we can be fairly certain that lymphoedema arises due to either surgical or radiation treatment or a combination of both. In past years lymphoedema was almost inevitable after radical mastectomy, but as surgical methods have changed over the past few years, this is now not so. However, with recent trends of limited surgery to the breast and axillary sampling, radiation therapy has become more radical in its aim to eradicate the disease, so we are still left with a possible problem of inadequate lymphatic drainage of the arm.

MANAGEMENT

Management of arm oedema can be divided into three aspects: prevention, active treatment of established cases, and palliative care.

Information about arm care remains a highly sensitive subject in the UK. Some surgeons feel that the patient has a right to be fully informed about the possibilities of arm oedema, whilst other surgeons say that such information is alarmist and unnecessary. It is worth noting that this latter group of doctors usually have no constructive advice to offer once their patient has lymphoedema. Whilst nurses cannot change attitudes overnight, they can learn a little about the subject so that more information can be offered to the patient.

Prevention

Prevention too is a controversial topic, as many surgeons either think that lymphoedema is inevitable or firmly believe that 'their patients don't get it'. The latter group of doctors may only follow-up their patients for a couple of years and then discharge them to the care of the GP, so they may never see the full extent of their patients who do get lymphoedema. Many of these patients are left to struggle on by themselves, so the true number of patients with this condition never comes to light. Often, without any specialised knowledge on the subject, GPs may say that nothing can be done, and placate the patient by saying that it is a 'small price to pay for a cure'.

Whilst in hospital, the patient who has undergone *any* type of breast surgery should be taught arm exercises which are designed to enable her to use her arm normally, and activities such as brushing her hair and changing her nightdress should be encouraged.

The nurse's role in prevention

Firstly, the nurse's role in most of the care of the arm and shoulder is that of aiding co-workers; that is the physiotherapist and surgeon, as they may have special instructions on each individual patient. Where this is not so, the nursing staff must then be guided by the physiotherapist.

An additional role is to encourage her patient to exercise her arm under the supervision of the physiotherapist. If the physiotherapist advises exercises to be done more than once a day, the nurse should ensure her patient follows these instructions. She can reassure the patient that the axillary stitches will come to no harm. Proper timing of analgesics (such as distalgesics), given half an hour before physiotherapy commences, will enable the patient to be relaxed and pain-free in order to take part in her exercise programme.

The outpatient nurse must be ready to offer continuing care of the arm and shoulder, and observe her patients who come for postoperative follow-up, so that appropriate referrals to physiotherapy can be made if shoulder and arm movements show any sign of deterioration.

A typical example of a 'Hand and Arm Care' scheme might include:

1 Use your arm as normally as possible, though heavier housework should not be undertaken for the first six weeks after your operation.

2 Avoid cuts, scratches, grazes, etc. to any part of the affected arm. Should any of these occur, wash the wound thoroughly with a suitable antiseptic solution. Observe for swelling and/or redness and contact your GP if this does not subside, so that appropriate treatment can begin immediately.

Initially if the woman has had a left mastectomy, she may experience a problem if driving a manual car. Activities such as knitting, typing, piano playing, etc. should not give rise to any problems.

Treatment of lymphodema

Established cases fall into two groups, active and palliative.

Active treatment may be indicated for a woman who is generally quite fit and disease free, and for whom the enlarged arm may be causing a degree of embarrassment. Quite apart from the heaviness of the arm she may find difficulty getting clothes to fit her, complaining bitterly that she is a size 14, whilst her arm is a size 16! Providing that she has a full range of movement of the shoulder there are two approaches to her problem.

The first is referral to the physiotherapist, who may be able to advise a course of external intermittent compression therapy, a pressure graded elasticated sleeve and isometric exercises (Fig. 12.1).

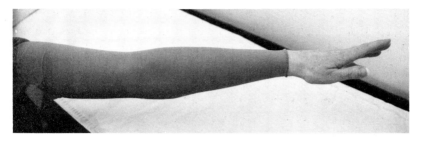

Fig. 12.1 A specially made elasticated pressured graded sleeve. (Photography courtesy of Jobst.)

The aim of all this is to reduce the size of the arm by gently squeezing the fluid back through the small lymphatic channels in the axilla. Other therapies include Faradism, bandaging, massage and arm elevation. Some successes have been reported by use of these methods, though the woman must be totally committed to the treatment programme set out by the physiotherapist. Other active methods of reducing the size of the limb include the use of diuretics, and advice on general weight loss if the patient is obese. The drawback of these methods is that the reduction in size must be held by a maintenance therapy, as the fluid will inevitably return within a few days of stopping the treatment. If this fact is not explained to the patient at the beginning of treatment, she may become extremely disheartened. Lymphangioplasty has been tried in several cases, though again the problem is only temporarily relieved, and the patient has the added problem of unsightly scars on her inner arm.

The second way of dealing with the woman's problem (if she does not wish to partake of the above programme) is to advise her about suitable styles of clothes which would help to conceal the enlarged arm (Fig. 12.2). Helpful hints on how to make a cuff larger, or how to insert a strip of material into the inside seam are also useful. Any sewing class would be able to teach her how to do this. (The Mastectomy Association also publishes an information sheet on how to alter sleeves.)

Palliation

When it comes to the care of the terminal patient with a swollen arm, the task of care falls to the nurse, both in the ward and the district.

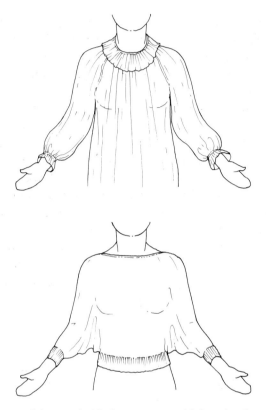

Fig. 12.2   Types of sleeve suitable for a woman with lymphoedema of the arm.

The cause of lymphoedema at this stage is usually a combination of surgery, radiotherapy and tumour involvement of the axilla, so the arm is likely to get progressively worse. Nodules which exudate lymph may be present, and require frequent dry dressings to absorb the fluid. Systemic chemotheraputic agents sometimes have a limited effect upon the speed upon which the deterioration takes place, but are not generally felt to improve matters. The aim is to keep the patient comfortable, by positioning the arm however she wishes — though it seems to be more beneficial to have the arm elevated and well supported on pillows. Some patients find a great deal of comfort by using Tubigrip, which should not be tight nor cause red marks to appear on the arm. Other patients may wish to continue to use their compression pump if they possess one.

None of the above will make much impact on the size of the swollen limb, but may give some temporary relief from the tightness and heaviness. They will almost certainly give emotional comfort to the patient, who will feel at least something is being attempted to ease the situation.

Strong sunlight should be avoided, as should excesses of heat and cold. If the skin is flaky and dry, it can be moisturised by suitable creams or oils, which may help to alleviate some of the tightness, though many women find the arm is too painful even for this simple measure to be of any help. Such women will almost certainly feel embarrassed or socially unacceptable with their large arm and will try to hide it away as much as possible when visitors arrive. The nurse by being sensitive to this can perhaps suggest the use of a pretty, long-sleeved dressing gown or bed jacket to wear. Attention to general morale is important — a lymphoedematous hand may not allow the patient to apply lipstick or face powder any more, nor hold a pen to write a simple thank you note.

EXERCISE

The lymph nodes in Evelyn's axilla have caused inadequate lymphatic drainage from her left arm. Consequently, she has developed slight lymphoedema.

1 What physical, psychological and social problems might result from this lymphoedema?

2 What nursing and medical methods might be employed to alleviate this condition?

Chapter 13
Specific Problems and Nursing Care: Local Spread and Metastatic Disease

Let us now examine the specific areas of spread from breast cancer, problems which can arise in patients with metastatic disease, and the actions which nurses can take to minimise and care for patients with these problems.

LOCAL SPREAD

Breast cancer can invade the areas around the chest wall and the mastectomy scar line even years after the operation was carried out. This is usually termed *local recurrence*. The main problems and nursing actions for this first type of spread are as follows:

Problem.   Pain at site of spread.
Action.   Give analgesia as prescribed and monitor its effectiveness. Discover which position is most comfortable for your patient and help the patient to get into the most comfortable positions.

Problem.   Possible infection due to skin breakdown at site of local spread.
Action.   Take frequent wound swabs to monitor progress.
Dress area as necessary using non-adherent dressing with cotton wool for protection and to absorb exudate.

Problem.   Possible offensive odour from breakdown of tissue at site of local spread.
Action.   Use charcoal pads on top of dressing to absorb odour.
Use 'nilodor' or other anti-odour device near her bed.
Encourage patient to use favourite perfume so that she is not constantly bothered by the smell.

Problem. Feelings of isolation and wanting to be alone because of the offensive odour.
Action. Help her realise that the charcoal dressings are lessening or removing the odour.
Encourage her to get dressed in ordinary clothes and to socialise with other patients especially at meal times or to watch television.

Local spread of disease can be excised surgically or treated by radiotherapy in some patients depending upon the extent of their previous surgery and whether or not they have had radiotherapy to that area in the past. Some specialist centres are excising badly fungating local recurrence lesions and applying a graft taken from abdominal omentum or latissimus dorsi, followed by a skin graft to the site. This is a palliative measure which does not attempt to cure the local recurrence but is done to improve quality of life by removing the offensive area and replacing it by non-offensive, healthy tissue.

METASTATIC DEPOSITS IN BONE

One of the most common places for breast cancer to spread is to bony areas. Any bony area can be affected including vertebrae, long bones of the legs and arms, the pelvis or the ribs. The site in which a bony lesion is discovered will greatly influence the types of problems and symptoms which the woman experiences. Pain is a problem which is often associated with secondary deposits in the bone and yet many people develop bone secondaries and remain pain free.

To understand the reason for this, one needs to recall some basic facts about the anatomy of bone. First of all, the sensory nerves in the bone are only located in the outer layer of bone called the *periosteum*. Patients with secondary bone deposits can have these lesions in parts of the bone other than the periosteum. These patients will not, on the whole, experience pain in these bones. Secondary bone deposits which do affect the periosteum are those which cause a tremendous amount of pain to the patient. As normal bone tissue is replaced by malignant tissue from breast cancer, the bone tissue breaks down. Two things can happen as the normal bone tissue disintegrates:

firstly, the chances of the bone weakening and eventually breaking are great; secondly, as bone tissue breaks down, huge amounts of calcium from the bone are released into the blood stream causing hypercalcaemia. This will be discussed later in this chapter.

The amount of pain and resulting immobility will depend upon the site of the secondary deposits — in other words, which bones are involved. The treatment for bone secondaries depends upon many factors which have been discussed in previous chapters. Radiotherapy is an effective way, in some patients, to remove the pain from the affected area, to stop the bone from breaking down further. Depending upon the age of the patient and the hormonal status and response of the tumour to hormone therapy, some type of endocrine treatment might be effective to treat bone secondaries.

Bone pain does not respond as well to strong narcotic analgesia as do other types of pain from cancer. Aspirin or aspirin mixed with other agents like paracetamol and Nepenthe are effective analgesic agents for patients with bone pain. The most important thing for nurses to remember when looking after patients with severe bone pain is that patients respond differently to different analgesia; it is the nurses' responsibility to monitor and record how well the pain is responding to the analgesia.

Problem.   Pain at site of bone secondary deposit.
Action.   Give the analgesia as prescribed by the doctor. Find out from the patient how it is working and look for facial or postural signs as to how it is working.

If bone deposit is in legs or spine:

Problem.   Immobility due to pain in back or legs.
Action.   This will depend upon size and severity of bone lesion. If it is safe for her to try to mobilise once the pain is under control then this must be discussed, encouraged and monitored by the nurse.
If it is safe to begin helping the patient to mobilise, start slowly with sitting on the side of the bed, then being lifted into a chair, progressing to partial weight-bearing with a nurse in support on either side; then gradually helping her to walk, first with crutches and

then unaided. Remember, the ability to increase mobility will depend upon pain control, gentle support and encouragement by nurses and her family.

In cases of severe bone deposits in legs and spine:

Problem.   Possible fracture of limb or vertebral collapse.
Action.   Your patient should not mobilise if fracture or vertebral collapse is possible.
Any movement to the patient must be carried out very carefully with support to the affected area.

Vertebral lesions are especially dangerous in that neurological damage can occur to the spine at the site of the deposit. Radiotherapy is usually commenced immediately and neurological examination and observations must be monitored to detect sensory or motor changes in the leg or trunk. Loss of neurological function will depend upon the part of the spine which has been damaged. Lumbar and sacral lesions can cause loss of movement and feeling to the legs and feet. Upper lumbar and thoracic vertebral lesions can lead to neurogenic bladder, urinary and faecal incontinence or constipation. Deposits in the cervical vertebrae can lead to loss of feeling and movement from the neck down (including the arms, legs and trunk) and can lead to quadriplegia.

Pain leads to extreme anxiety, especially in a woman who has gone through other forms of treatment in the past such as mastectomy, and has had to cope with cancer for a long time. The immobility that accompanies pain from bone secondaries is also a very depressing thing for a woman to face. There is a need for sensitivity on the part of the nursing staff and' a willingness to encourage the patient to talk about feelings and frustrations until palliative measures to relieve the pain and bring about a return to mobility can be effected.

Hypercalcaemia

In the breakdown of bone tissue by secondary deposits, calcium is released in large quantities into the bloodstream. This is an extremely serious and dangerous complication of bone breakdown and, although the symptoms and manifestations of hypercalcaemia can be treated, unless the cause of the hypercalcaemia is treated, death will occur.

A certain level of calcium is required by the body to maintain neuromuscular excitability. If calcium levels are too high, as in this instance, many parts of the body are affected and many symptoms will occur. As the raised calcium levels are circulated in the blood, the kidneys develop a greatly increased tubular reabsorption rate for calcium. This is the body's attempt to remove the excess calcium from the blood by excreting it in the urine. In excreting this excess calcium, a large amount of water is also excreted. As this excess water is lost in urine, considerable amounts of sodium and potassium are lost as well. Neuromuscular excitability is impaired and the most noticeable manifestation of this is atony of the gut leading to constipation. This in turn causes nausea and vomiting which increases the likelihood of dehydration.

A raised serum calcium level inhibits the action of antidiuretic hormone in the pituitary gland. Because of this, even more water is lost in urine and a situation not unlike diabetes insipidus ensues where the patient suffers from polydipsia (excessive thirst) as well as polyuria (excessive urinary output). Raised calcium levels lead to toxicity to the nervous system, causing lethargy, drowsiness, confusion and (if left untreated) coma and death. Hypercalcaemia causes the following problems in patients with bone secondaries:

1   Constipation.
2   Extreme thirst.
3   Excess urinary output leading to dehydration and electrolyte imbalance.
4   Lethargy leading to confusion or coma or death.
5   Nausea and vomiting.

The medical staff will treat this condition in two ways: firstly, by treating the symptoms with intravenous replacement of fluids and electrolytes; secondly by lowering the level of calcium in the blood by giving intravenous mithramycin (which lowers serum calcium levels) and corticosteroids, and by halting the spread of bone secondary tumour through the use of radiotherapy, hormone therapy or chemotherapy.

The nursing staff will be responsible for keeping the patient safe and comfortable; carefully watching over intravenous therapy; seeing that total hygiene needs are being met with sensitive care to the mouth (especially after vomiting has occurred); checking elimination needs (in view of constipation and polyuria); and observing and recording any changes in levels of consciousness, of urinary output, nausea/vomiting and thirst.

SECONDARY DEPOSITS IN THE BRAIN

In the course of its systemic spread breast cancer may lead to the formation of secondary deposits in the brain. The symptoms which occur will depend to a great extent on the location of the lesion in the brain. Brain secondary deposits can occur in the occipital (posterior) region of the brain which can affect vision. Other brain lesions, depending upon their location, may cause any of the following problems or symptoms:

1 Ataxia and unsteadiness on feet.
2 Speech problems where the patient knows which words she is trying to say, but what comes out when she tries to speak is unintelligible.
3 Inability to communicate through writing or reading due to not being able to form the words on paper as she has them in her mind, or inability to recognise words written on paper.
4 Hemiplegia or hemiparesis.
5 Headaches.
6 Personality change.
7 Nausea and vomiting due to raised intracranial pressure.

THE NURSE'S ROLE

Depending upon the severity of the symptoms, the patient and her family may be extremely anxious about these problems and symptoms. If communication difficulties are part of the presenting symptoms the woman feels an almost unbearable sense of frustration and anger at not being able to communicate and make herself understood. Whatever the presenting problem, the nurse's role is to identify the problems as they arise, observe for signs of improvement or change, and develop the type of relationship with her patient and the family which will make it easier to communicate with them and alleviate their anxiety.

Treatment for brain secondaries is palliative. The object is not to cure the patient at this stage in the disease but to relieve symptoms and improve quality of life. Hormone therapy and chemotherapy have little place in the palliative treatment of brain secondaries because few of these drugs cross the blood-brain barrier. This means that although we can inject drugs into a vein or give tablets which eventually reach the bloodstream, the protective mechanism in the blood vessels leading to the brain is such that it does not allow these drugs to enter the cerebral blood supply. Patients with brain secondaries who present with any of the above problems are therefore treated with radiotherapy.

In many of these patients the symptom relief is quite good, thus improving the patients' ability to go home and live relatively symptom-free for the remainder of their lives. The patient and family must be made aware that radiotherapy to the brain will result in alopecia. This can prove to be a devastating side-effect to the woman especially if she has previously faced a period of alopecia when receiving chemotherapy in the past. Again, the nurse must play a supportive role, providing practical assistance in the form of ordering a wig and encouraging the woman to concentrate on other aspects of her femininity such as using attractive head scarves, make-up and clothing.

SECONDARY LIVER DISEASE

It is common for patients with breast cancer to develop metastatic deposits in the liver. Depending upon the severity and size of the secondary tumour any of the following problems may occur in patients with liver secondaries:

1   Yellow tinge to the skin (jaundice) due to blockage of bile-producing cells of the liver.

2   Itching/flaking skin due to jaundice.

3   A further change in body image from ascites if liver damage is severe.

4   Dyspnoea due to pressure of ascites on diaphragm.

5   Nausea, vomiting and anorexia due to ascites pressing on the stomach.

6   Constipation due to absence of bile entering the large intestine and to pressure on intestines from ascites.

7   Possible skin breakdown and pressure sores due to flaking skin and bile deposits from jaundice.

8   Pain and discomfort from ascites.

The amount and extent of nursing care which will be needed by women with liver metastases from breast cancer primary tumours will depend upon the severity of the liver involvement. Special attention is needed to keep skin healthy and intact since skin breakdown is a real possibility in jaundiced patients. Nutritional needs are often a challenge in patients with liver secondaries because of anorexia and of the change in metabolic processes due to malfunctioning of the liver. This is made even more difficult by the nausea, vomiting and anorexia which accompanies liver metastases. Treatment of liver metastases is by abdominal paracentesis if ascites is present. The ascitic fluid is drained off through a cannula inserted into the abdominal cavity. When fluid has finished draining, chemotherapeutic agents such as Bleomycin or Thiotepa can be inserted into the abdominal cavity to try to decrease the liver deposits and prevent recurrence of ascites. Even with this treatment, there is a high likelihood of ascites recurring at a later time. Systemic treatment can be given in the form of intravenous chemotherapy but the prognosis at this stage is extremely poor.

THE DETECTION OF METASTATIC DEPOSITS

After a patient has undergone some form of primary treatment for breast cancer, usually involving surgery and/or radiotherapy, follow-up clinical check-ups will continue monitoring the progress of the patient. At each visit investigations will be carried out to observe the sites of likely metastatic spread, such as the bone and the liver. Blood tests will be carried out to observe blood count (which may alter if the disease is spreading to the bone marrow) and serum calcium levels (to detect bone breakdown from metastases). Radioactive scanning of bones may also be carried out. This involves an intravenous injection of a small dose of a radioactive isotope which is picked up by the bones. X-rays are taken of the entire skeletal system and areas of greater radioisotope uptake can be detected. In this way bone secondaries can be detected when they are very small even before they are clinically evident. Ultrasonic scanning of the liver can also be carried out to detect early evidence of liver deposits. The results of tests such as these plus good clinical examination will allow the patient to be treated before the metastatic disease becomes clinically evident and the problems become too severe to be dealt with. The decision as to what treatment is often a difficult one but, at this stage of the patient's disease, the object of treatment is to reduce or prevent problematic symptoms and to give patients a reasonable quality of life. Patients need time and space to sort out whatever life they have left, to prepare themselves and their families for their death, and to enjoy whatever time they have left as pain-free and symptom-free as is possible.

EXERCISE

Evelyn has now developed pain in her lower back and left leg. A bone scan confirms that this pain is being caused by metastatic deposits at both these sites.

1   What other problems might be caused by these bone metastases?
2   What observations would lead the nursing staff to suspect that Evelyn might be developing hypercalcaemia?
3   What nursing measures might be taken to alleviate the symptoms (and subsequent anxiety) brought by hypercalcaemia?

Appendix 1
The Mastectomy Association

The Mastectomy Association was founded in 1973 in order to give advice and information on the non-medical aspects of postmastectomy needs. The aim of the Association is to complement the medical and nursing care already done in many hospitals and clinics throughout the UK. As a registered charity (assisted financially by the Department of Health and Social Security) there are a number of services freely available for both patient and nurse to use.

Over the years the Association has built up a comprehensive network of volunteer helpers who have undergone mastectomy in the past. These women are willing to listen and talk to the new client about their non-medical needs, and may be able to offer advice and encouragement if needed.

Both hospital and community nurses can obtain literature from the Mastectomy Association simply by contacting them directly. 'Sample' packs of literature include the Health Education Councils booklet *Living with the loss of a breast,* as well as an up-to-date list of stockists selling suitable bras, swimwear and other fashion wear. There is also an exhibition of breast forms and fashion wear suitable for post mastectomy wear at the Association Head Office, where both nurse and client will be made welcome.

The Mastectomy Association has also formed links with many hospitals throughout the country and has the advantage that staff are kept up-to-date with new non-medical developments which may be of help to their patient. The staff at the Mastectomy Association will be pleased to deal with any enquiries from either client or nurse and are there to help. Their address is 26 Harrison Street, London WC1H 8JG (Telephone 01-837 0908).

Appendix 2
Counselling Organisations

The Mastectomy Association
26 Harrison Street
London WC1H 8JG

01 837 0908

Women's National Cancer Control Campaign
1 South Audley Street
London W1Y 5DQ

01 499 7532/4

Cancer Help Centre
Grove House
Cornwallis Road
Clifton
Bristol BS8 4PC

0272 743216

This organisation is a unique one that uses physical, psychological and spiritual means to treat patients with cancer.

Cancerlink
46A Pentonville Road
London N1 9HF

01 833 2451

This organisation is a charity which provides information for cancer patients and their families and initiates and supports cancer self-help groups.

British Association for Counselling
1a Little Church Street
Rugby
Warwickshire

Appendix 3
Directory of Apparel/Prostheses Suppliers

This list is a compilation of one issued by the Mastectomy Association with several additions. For updates of this list contact the Mastectomy Association (address in Appendix 2).

AVON	**Phone No.**
Ellis Son & Paramore, 11 George St, Bath	0225 63065
Dorothy Rogers, 85 Hill Rd, Clevedon	0272 872836
Mary's Norton House, High St, Midsomer Norton	0761 412196
Great Expectations, 8 The Centre, Weston Super Mare	0934 418034
Surgical & Ortho. App. Ltd, 20 Filton Rd, Horfield, Bristol	0272 44919

BEDFORDSHIRE	
Contessa, 13 West Arcade, Bedford	0234 55434
Contessa, 120 Dunstable Rd, Luton	0582 20765
Croxfords Ltd, Market Sq, Leighton Buzzard	

BERKSHIRE	
Thames Valley Medical, 118A Chatham St, Reading	0734 595835
Debenhams of Reading	
Heelas of Reading	
Owen & Owen, 155 High St, Slough	75 26942
Contessa, 66 Broadway, Bracknell	0344 59622
Contessa, 68A High St, Maidenhead	93 24077
Contessa, 8 Denmark St, Wokingham	983 785166
W.L. Daniel, Peascod St, Windsor	95 62106

BUCKINGHAMSHIRE	
Ladyfair, 1 Station Parade, Beaconsfield	04946 3408
Contessa, 24B White Hart St, High Wycombe	0494 22954
Contessa, 10 The Concourse, Brunel Centre, Milton Keynes	0908 72810

CAMBRIDGESHIRE	
Eaden Lilley, Market St, Cambridge	0223 358822

CHESHIRE

Contessa, 8 Victoria Centre, Crewe	0270 21640
Contessa, 48 Mill St, Macclesfield	0625 617816

CLEVELAND

P.C. Peacocks, 183 Borough Rd, Middlesborough	0642 247900
Mrs J. Parkinson, 5 Truro Drive, Hartlepool	0429 870359
Finnegans, 10 Yarm Lane, Stockton on Tees	0642 607796

CORNWALL

W.J. Roberts, Boscawen St, Truro	
Mrs. Poole, 13 Trelawny Rd, St. Austell (Home fittings)	0726 3008
Hendra (Chemist), Lemon St, Truro	

CUMBRIA

Ellis Son & Paramore, 4 Frith Drive, St Bees	094 685 369

DERBY

Contessa, 40 Peters St, Derby	0332 380162
Ellis Son & Paramore, 111 London Rd, Derby	0332 44147
Mrs I. Buckley, 'Bodycare', 15 High St, Alfreton	077383 2882
Mrs M. Thompson, Chesterfield (Camp/Strodex-home fittings)	0246 852647

DEVON

W.H. Chope, 13 High St, Bideford	023 72 2091
Plymouth & S. Devon Co-op, Derry's Cross, Plymouth	0752 66280

DORSET

Beales, Old Christchurch Rd, Bournemouth	0202 22022
Weymouth & Dist. Co-op, Westham Rd, Weymouth	03057 83101
Contessa, 690/2 Christchurch Rd, Boscombe	0202 34851
Beasleys, 124 Poole Rd, Westbourne, Bournemouth	0202 764633
Beasleys, 4 Kingland Crescent, Poole	02013 4738
G.E. Bridge, 125 Old Christchurch Rd, Bournemouth	0202 20521
Valerie Milward, 51 Carbery Ave, Southbourne, Bournemouth	0202 429004

DURHAM

Northern Surgical, Post House Wynd, Darlington	0325 64699

ESSEX

Sarah (Corsetière), 29 London Rd, Barking	
Bertha Leeds, 29 Crouch St, Colchester	0206 76914
Contessa, 11 Little Walk, Harlow	0279 417415
Sarah (Corsetière), 102 South St, Romford	
E. Robson, 279 London Rd, Westcliffe on Sea	0702 49169
Shirley Shawe, 26 Inglehurst Gardens, Ilford	01 550 4575

GLOUCESTERSHIRE

Contessa, 156 High St, Cheltenham	0242 39449
Contessa, 40 Dyer St, Cirencester	0285 4335
Contessa, 2 Market Way, Eastgate Centre, Gloucester	0452 416136
Contessa, c/o Wm. McIlroys, King St, Stroud	04536 4232

HAMPSHIRE

Contessa, 75 High St, Andover	0264 4005
Contessa, 37A West St, Fareham	03292 80477
Contessa, 72 Queensmead, Farnborough	94 42687
Longley's, 335/7 Fleet Rd, Fleet	9484 3808
Contessa, 92/3 High St, Gosport	07017 83391
Contessa, 11 High St, Lymington	0590 72458
Contessa, 92 High St, Shirley, Southampton	0703 771192
Contessa, 2 The Precinct, London Rd, Waterlooville	07014 2676
Longley's, 15 Church St, Basingstoke	0256 21290
Mrs Patricia Longley, Winchester (Home fittings)	0962 69931
Camp Masters & Lindseys, 110 Elmgrove, Southsea	0705 697411
Landports, Commercial Rd, Portsmouth	
Debenhams, Queensway, Southampton	
Walton's, 85 Queen St, Portsmouth	0705 25153

HEREFORD

Contessa, 15 Commercial St, Hereford	0432 54561

HERTFORDSHIRE

Contessa, 3 Market Place, Hatfield	07072 64670
Contessa, 230 Marlowes, Hemel Hempstead	0442 51588
Contessa, 19 The Churchyard, Hitchin	0462 2172
Contessa, 3 Commerce Way, Letchworth	04626 3408
Contessa, 2 George St, Albans	0727 53664
Contessa, 29 Queensway, Stevenage	0438 52308
Contour, 12 Wigmores South, Welwyn Garden City	07073 27171
Mrs M. Hamilton, 20 Cross Rd, Oxhey, Watford (Home fittings)	92 34827
Clements, 29 The Parade, Watford	92 44222

HUMBERSIDE

Binns, House of Fraser, Paragon Sq., Hull	0482 26951

ISLE OF WIGHT

Pack & Culliford, Union St, Ryde	

KENT

Contessa, 160 Broadway, Bexleyheath	01 303 1142
Gadsby's, 27 High St, Sidcup	01 300 2029
Contessa, 86 High St, Sittingbourne	0795 72454
Contessa, 20 Calverley Rd, Tunbridge Wells	0892 26751

Townsend Ltd, 175 Ashford Rd, Canterbury   0227 62713
Allders of Bromley, Market Sq., Bromley
Allders of Chatham, High St, Chatham
Debenhams of Canterbury (fitter Mon/Tue/Thurs)
Horton's Corsetières, 42 Monson Rd, Tunbridge Wells   0892 27401
Army & Navy, Bromley
The Corset Shop, Market Sq., Bromley   01 460 3470
Rita Richards, Town Sq., Erith
Rita Richards, Nuxley Rd, Belvedere

LANCASHIRE
Blackburn Co-op
Corbra, 3 Water St, Accrington
Ida Walton, 23 Waterloo Rd, Blackpool   0253 42231
Suzanne, Arndale House, King St, Lancaster   0524 2856
Beasleys, 126 Victoria Rd, Cleveleys, Blackpool   0253 852043
Contessa, 95 St. James St, Burnley   0282 26663
Contessa, 8 Fishergate Walk, St. Georges Centre, Preston   0772 51926
Slater & Co., 8 Caunce St, Blackpool   0253 20745
Debenhams of Blackburn
Body Lines, Tower Centre Shopping Precinct, Blackburn
Bellman's Corsetry, 60 Drake St, Rochdale

LEICESTERSHIRE
Carole Molyneux, Francis St, Stoneygate, Leicester   0533 709252
Valerie, 4A High St, Oakham   0572 55900

LONDON
Bradleys, 26 Marylebone High St, W1   01 935 1216
Bradleys, 83 Knightsbridge, SW1   01 235 2902
Contour, 2 Hans Rd, Knightsbridge, SW3   01 589 9293
Dickins & Jones, Regent St, W1   01 734 7070
Petite Professional Services, 17 Newman Passage, W1   01 580 8951
Alfred Cox, 106 Whitechapel Rd, E1   01 247 1178
Donald Rose, 36 George St, Portman Square, W1   01 935 4346
Downe Bros., 32 New Cavendish St, W1   01 486 3611
A.B. Ockenden, 84 Park Way, NE1   01 485 0136
Camp Masters & Lindseys, 116 Tower Bridge Rd, SE1   01 237 3195
Contessa, 14 Topsfield Parade, Crouch End, N8   01 348 0518
Arding & Hobbs, Clapham Junction, SW11
Whiteleys of Bayswater, Queensway, W2
Christina Berry, N13 (Home fittings)   01 886 7633
Army & Navy Stores, Victoria St, SW1   01 834 1234
Rose Lewis, 40 Knightsbridge, SW1   01 235 6885
Chiesmans of Lewisham   01 852 4321
Barkers of Kensington   01 937 5432
Rigby & Peller, 12 South Molton St, W1   01 629 6708

MANCHESTER

Contessa, 9 Grafton Mall, Altrincham	061 928 5339
Contessa, 5 The Mall, Sale	061 969 5208
Prince & Fletcher, Bonding House, 26 Blackfriars St,	
Salford	061 834 5573
T.S. Shannon, 59 Bradford St, Bolton	0204 21789
Mrs Lilian Mason, 7 Monument Rd, Wigan	0942 45730
Elizabeth, 14 New Parade, Rectory Gardens, Cheadle	061 428 4707
Kendal Milne, Deansgate, Manchester	

MERSEYSIDE

Camp Masters & Lindseys, 15 Moss St, Liverpool	051 207 1675
Contessa, 13 Wallasey Rd, Wallasey	051 639 9844

MIDDLESEX

Lilian Read, 39 Burnt Oak Broadway, Edgward	01 205 8270
Contessa, 434 Greenford Rd, Greenford	01 578 1160
Contessa, 35 King St Parade, Twickenham	01 892 1790
Contessa, 51 High St, Wealdstone	01 427 0641

NORFOLK

Barbara Branch, 52 Lowestoft Rd, Gorleston on Sea	0493 62533
John Lewis, All Saints Green, Norwich	
Garlands of Norwich, London St, Norwich	
Butchers, Swan Lane, Norwich	

NORTHAMPTONSHIRE

T.D. Roper, 3 Derngate, Northampton	
Contessa, 39 Corporation St, Corby	05366 3909
Contessa, 63A Abington St, Northampton	0604 38346
Contessa, 32 Market St, Wellingborough	0933 76628
Kettering Surgical Appliances, 55 Ambush St, Northampton	0604 57179
Lane Orthopaedics, 8 Bridge St, Northampton	0604 32069

OXFORDSHIRE

Spencer (Surgical) Ltd, Spencer House, Britannia Rd,	
Banbury	0295 57301
Contessa, 10 Church Lane, Banbury	0295 4205
Contessa, 13 The Square, Cowley	0865 778877

SHROPSHIRE

Peterwood, 1 Willow St, Oswestry	0691 59225
Contessa, Market Square, Wellington, Telford	0952 47822

SOMERSET

The Corsetry Cottage, 19 Bath Place, Taunton	

STAFFORDSHIRE
Donald Wardle & Son, 20 West Precinct, Hanley, Stoke on
    Trent   0782 25160

SUFFOLK
T.W. Rose, 60 St. Matthews St, Ipswich   0473 58508

SURREY
Contour, 1021 Whitgift Centre, Croydon   01 681 1153
Contessa, 2 Town Hall Buildings, Farnham   01 681 1153
Dickins & Jones, George St, Richmond
W. Haslett, Church St, Weybridge   97 42335
Contessa, 32 Obelisk Way, Camberley   82 29665
Contessa, 8 Tunsgate Sq, Guildford   0483 69168
Contessa, 11 Bridge St, Leatherhead   03723 72371
Contessa, 40 The Centre, Hepworth Way, Walton on
    Thames   962 21858
Contessa, 5 Wolsey Walk, Woking   04862 61376
Pillow Talk, 65A High St, Reigate   74 40202
Bentalls, Kingston on Thames   01 546 1001
Fininley Ltd, 61 London Rd, West Croydon   01 688 2017
Allders of Croyden
Allders, High St, Sutton
Army & Navy, Camberley

SUSSEX
Contessa, 39 Queens Sq, Crawley   0293 24912
Contessa, 55 London Rd, East Grinstead   0342 21661
Madame Greenaway, 40/40A Robertson St, Hastings   0424 436425
Contessa, 54/6 South Rd, Haywards Heath   0444 412171
Contessa, 27 Swan Walk, Horsham   0403 68466
Contessa, 30 George St, Hove   0273 772575
Contessa, 133 The Street, Rustington   09062 2787
Genevieve, 18 The Martlets, Crawley   0293 21433
A.B. Ockenden, 45/7 Teville Rd, Worthing   0903 39661
Joan Crocker, 42 Goring Rd, Worthing   0903 504603
Debenhams of Worthing
Moran's (Army & Navy), Chichester
Chesterfield, Western Road, Brighton
Camp Masters & Lindsey's, Queen St, Hastings   0424 42005

TYNE & WEAR
P.C. Peacocks, 1A St. Thomas St, Newcastle on Tyne   0632 29917

WARWICKSHIRE
Contessa, 8 Manning Walk, Rugby Centre, Rugby   0788 75816

WEST MIDLANDS

Co-op, Orchard House, The Precinct, Coventry	
Salt & Son, 220 Corporation St, Birmingham	021 236 2235
Dudley Surgical Appliances, 8 Dudley Port, Tipton	021 557 4204
R. Taylor, 29 Woodwards Rd, Pleck, Walsall	0922 27601
Wardens, 83/5 High St, Solihull	021 704 1161
Contessa, 19 Shelton Sq, Coventry	0203 25684
Contessa, 25 Bradford Mall, Saddler Centre, Walsall	0922 646561
Contessa, 12 Central Arcade, Mander Centre, Wolverhampton	0902 710010
Contessa, 29 The Precinct, Halesowen	021 550 7286
D.F. Hartland, 32a Queen St, Wolverhamton	0902 23512
Feminellas, 32 Market St, Stourbridge	

WILTSHIRE

Sarah (Corsetière), 36 Catherine St, Salisbury

WORCESTERSHIRE

Contessa, 125 High St, Bromsgrove	0527 71455
Contessa, 36 Bridge St, Evesham	0386 45718
Contessa, 20 The Bullring, Kidderminster	0562 746747
Contessa, 11 New Walk, Redditch	0527 67190

YORKSHIRE

L.S.B. Orthopaedics, Whitehall Rd, Farnley, Leeds	0532 792094
H.W. Poole, New York Rd (and Albion St), Leeds	0532 33045
Ellis Son & Paramore, 109 Devonshire St, Sheffield	0742 79141
Contessa, 27 Queensway, Keighley	0535 63228
Chapmans Corsetières, 20 County Arcade, Leeds	0532 456614
Contessa, 50 Northgate, Wakefield	0924 378380
Mary Freemantle, 37 Cleveland St, Doncaster	
Branded Lines, 2 High St, Skipton	
W.P. Brown, 21 Davygate, York	0904 54698
York Co-op, 22 George Hudson St, York	0904 22052
M. & J. Surgical Stores, 3 Colliergate, York	0904 26623

SCOTLAND

Salt & Son Ltd., 104 West George St, Glasgow	041 331 1643
Ellis Son & Paramore, 17 Commercial St, Dundee	0382 21593
Ellis Son & Paramore, 29 Innes St, Inverness	0463 36691
Anne Cole, The Corset Shop, 62 Queensberry St, Dumfries	0387 4255
Draffens of Dundee, Nethergate, Dundee	
The Chiffonier, 98 Morningside Rd, Edinburgh	
Katherine Henderson, 246 Kilmarnock Road, Glasgow	

WALES — GLAMORGAN

Madame Foner, 222 High St, Swansea	0792 53868
Allders, 8/9 Working St, Cardiff	

WALES — GWYNEDD

Peterwood, 213 High St, Bangor	0248 55567
Peterwood, Sheffield House, Ancaster Sq, Llanrwst	0492 640498
Peterwood, 107 High St, Porthmadog	0766 2141

WALES — CLWYD

Peterwood, 1/3 Crown Sq, Denbigh	074571 2561
Peterwood, 11 Tower Gardens, High St, Holywell	0352 710841
Contessa, 25 Daniel Owen Centre, Mold	0352 3168
Peterwood, 54 High St, Prestatyn	07456 6436
Peterwood, 15A Clwyd St, Ruthin	08242 2735

CHANNEL ISLANDS

Voisin & Co., King St, St. Helier, Jersey

MANUFACTURERS' ADDRESSES

Makers of breast prostheses:

Camp, Northgate House, Staple Gardens, Winchester, Hampshire

Donovan and Hanson Ltd, Abella House, Longden Road, Shrewsbury, Shropshire

Ellis Son and Paramore, Spring Street Works, Sheffield S38 P13

Kettering Surgical Appliances Ltd, 5 Harleston Road, St James', Northampton NN5 5LH

Remploy Ltd, Russ Street, Broad Plain, Bristol BS2 0HJ

Spenco Medical (UK) Ltd, Tanyard Lane, Steyning, West Sussex BN4 3RJ

Makers of mastectomy brassières and breast prostheses:

Spencer Surgical Supplies, Spencer House, Britannia Road, Banbury OX16 8DP

Makers of temporary breast prostheses (comfie):

Torplay, 3 Spinney Close, St Leonards, Ringwood BH24 2RB

Makers of elastic pressure sleeves and intermittent pressure therapy machines:

Huntleigh Medical Ltd, Bilton Way, Dallow Road, Luton LU1 1UU

Jobst (UK) Ltd, Service Centre, 17 Wigmore Street, London W1H 9LA

Jobst (Ireland) Ltd, Industrial Estate, Thurles, Co. Tipperary, Republic of Ireland

Pan Med Development Ltd, Edison Road, Churchfield, Salisbury SP2 7NU

E. Sallis Ltd, Vernon Works, Waterford Street, Basford, Nottingham

RELATED ADDRESSES

For guidelines about supplying breast forms:

Department of Health and Social Security, Block 1, Government Buildings, Warbreck Hill Road, Blackpool

Health Education Council, 78 New Oxford Street, London WC1 1AH

Index